A DOG ABROAD

One Man and his Dog Journey into
the Heart of Europe

Bruce Fogle

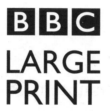

LARGE
PRINT

First published 2007
by Ebury Press
This Large Print edition published 2008
by BBC Audiobooks Ltd
by arrangement with
Ebury Press

Hardcover ISBN: 978 1 408 41379 1
Softcover   ISBN: 978 1 408 41380 7

British Library Cataloguing in Publication Data available

Printed and bound in Great Britain by
Antony Rowe, Chippenham, Wiltshire

CONTENTS

ACKNOWLEDGEMENTS

I come from a large, extended family. My mother was the youngest of ten, my father the second youngest of eight and almost all of these people not only continued to live near each other after they married, they continued to look upon their siblings and their spouses as best friends. That closeness, that natural ease of affection, percolated down to their children, to my generation. Until I left the close embrace of 'the family' when I moved away to university, all my best friends were first cousins.

A few of my cousins moved away from Toronto, to Quebec, Alberta, New Brunswick, California or Georgia, but we kept in touch and when I told some of them of my plans to drive through the Baltic States, then down through Poland to Slovakia, they responded with a wealth of interest and family information.

On my mother's side, Erik Newton in California sent me his 32-page highly illustrated family history of the Breslin clan, including photos I'd never seen of my great-great-grandfather, born in 1801, and my great-grandfather, born in 1835.

My Fogle cousins in Toronto, Diane Silver, Francie Hellen, Eleanor Loebel and Carolyn Schwartz, and more distant relatives in Glasgow, Harvey Bernard and Audrey Goodman, provided new (at least new to me) information about the Bernard and Fogle families. When all the bits and pieces were joined up, we were surprised by just how much information we held but didn't know we had. Thanks to all of you.

European friends and acquaintances were wonderfully generous with advice and information both for Macy and for me, and I'm grateful to Simon and Nel Roos in the Netherlands, Ruth Ragna Axen, Hilmar-Lutz and Elizabeth Poser in Germany, Charlotte Kristensen in Denmark, Kristina and Lars Gustafsson, Mats Olsson, Erika, Ulla and Ake Hedhammar, and Katarina Sjostrom in Sweden, Mati Kaal and Tiu Viires in Estonia and Simonas Dovidavicius, Arturas Abromavicius and Dovile Abromaviciute in Lithuania. Thanks to Mark Winer in London for providing translations of tombstones in Finland and Poland and to Peter Kertesz in London, my family's dentist for 30 years, for telling me about his upbringing in Hungary. Tom Lozar in Montreal offered terrific advice and information on Slovenia. Thank you.

It sounds precious to say so but it's undeniably true that I have another family to be grateful for; the people I work with. They certainly have stick-to-it-iveness. Some have been working with me for over 25 years. Simon Lewi, Veronica Aksmanovic, Ashley McManus, Suzi Gray, Hilary Hayward and Hester Small, you know I mean it when I say you're a wonderful group of people. You, and The Chief, my wife Julia, created time and space to let Macy and me enjoy our travels. To you all, thanks for your indulgence.

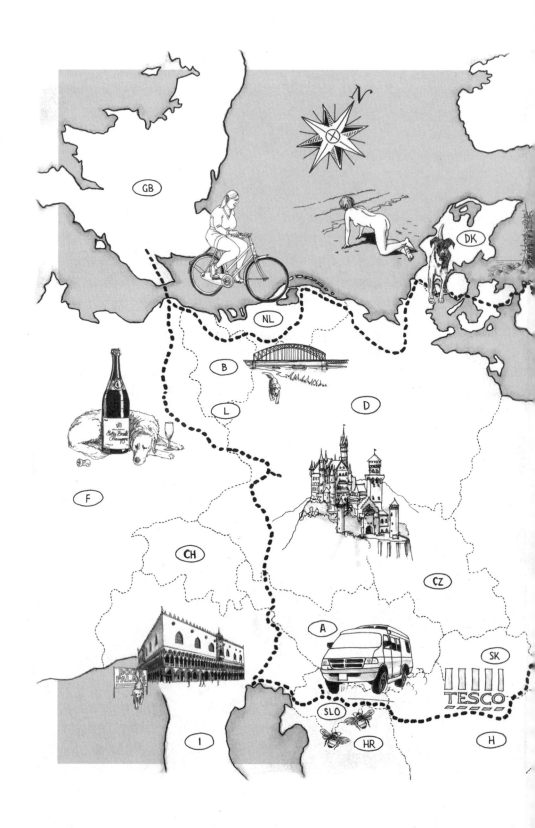

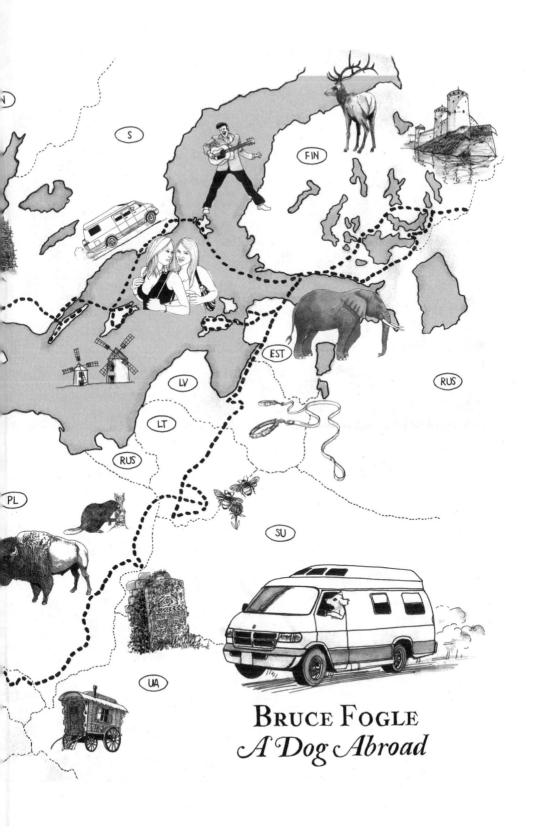

BRUCE FOGLE
A Dog Abroad

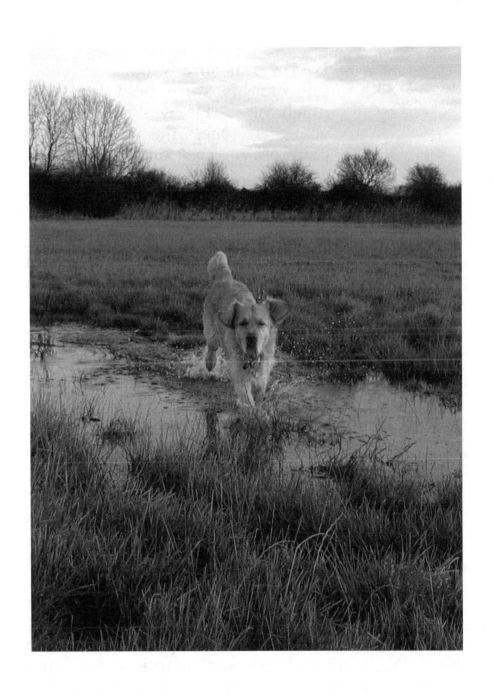

PREAMBLE

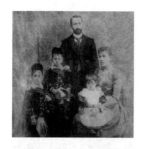 By the time my father wanted to tell me his story he'd forgotten much of it. He was nearing 100 years of age, the last of his generation, the only keeper of what would soon be lost memories, and now those stories were frayed and unreliable. 'I was born at 46 Ibrox Park Road, Glasgow, Scotland,' he offered without being asked, as I sat with him during his last weeks of life. Scotland was certainly an ongoing presence in his mind. There was pride in his Scottish heritage. It's no accident that my older brother's name is Robert, mine is Bruce and our first dog, a Scottish terrier, was named Angus.

Of course, I knew about the Fogle family's Scottish connection and not just from my father's and especially my grandmother's Glaswegian burr, nor simply from family photos of his older brothers in full Highland regalia as young boys or the pictures of my dad, in his twenties, playing the bagpipes. Cousins who were more interested than I had traced records of the ship on which the Fogle family had emigrated from Scotland to Canada in 1909. I knew that when he was a boy in Ottawa, my father routinely corresponded with a Scottish cousin, Tommy Bernard, who sent him sprigs of Scottish heather and who, in turn, received from my father, pressed crimson maple leaves and postcards written on birch bark. I know this because when I first visited Glasgow in 1964 Tommy showed me the stamped postcards he'd saved.

2

I also knew that the Fogles and my grandmother's Bernard family were not Scottish at all. They came from a mysterious, almost mythical place that my father said was called 'Kovna Gaberna'. He never knew exactly where that was, and never asked.

Last year, one of my cousins, Ros, gave her son Erik a mouth swab for his fortieth birthday. Erik was fascinated and intrigued with his family's heritage, and DNA, salvaged from the swab, provided him with what the lab called a 'personal genetic analysis'. Surprised by some of the results, Erik emailed them all to me, together with a list of questions. When I saw them I was surprised too. One of his strongest 'native population matches'— the geographical region that produced some of his most significant ancestral influence—was Strathclyde in Scotland, yet like my father, Erik isn't Scottish. Erik's ancestral origins are, like mine, partly in 'Kovna Gaberna'.

'What's up?' he asked.

Erik's personal genetic analysis produced a further anomaly. In the results, the world is divided into 23 distinct genetic regions, and he'd expected 'North-west European' to be his dominant genetic heritage but it wasn't. Nor was 'Eastern European' or 'Mediterranean'. 'Finno-Ugrian' was. A goodly proportion of Erik's genetic mother lode originated in the people who settled in Finland and Estonia. (Hungarians are usually counted as 'Finno-Ugrians' but in these results Hungarians fell into a separate category.)

*　　　*　　　*

3

This much I know: Kovna certainly isn't in Finland. 'Kovno' is the Russian name for the modern Lithuanian city of Kaunas, and Kovno Guberniya is the Imperial Russian province of Kovno—roughly present-day Lithuania. My father's parents, JR Fogle and Leah Bernard, were both born in Lithuania when it was part of the Russian Empire. My grandfather JR (for John Ralph, but originally Jacob Raphael) moved to Scotland in the 1880s as a very young boy with his parents and siblings. My grandmother arrived later, in 1893 when she was 17 years old, as a bride for JR, who was by then a student at Manchester University. They married the following year, then moved to Canada 16 years later.

Erik's research into his family's history and his curious genetic findings have triggered a nascent curiosity in me, a desire to know more about the place my parents' families emerged from, and to find out more about the rest of 'Eastern Europe'.

*   *   *

So I decided that now is the time to travel to the Baltic and beyond, through lands that western Europeans seldom visit, to go north-east through Scandinavia to the Russian border of Finland, then down along the distant rim of the expanded European Union, through Estonia (whose population shares a Finno-Ugrian heritage with the Finns), Latvia, Lithuania, Poland, Slovakia, and Hungary, finally emerging into Slovenia before heading back to the familiar territory of Italy. I'll take in not only the regions where my Fogle relatives lived, but also south-east Poland

and Slovakia—close to, or actually through, the lands where my mother's ancestors were once based. For most of my life the majority of that route has been a 'no-go' area, 'the communist bloc'.

*　　*　　*

There's a more pragmatic reason why now is the time to travel. Until last year, when the UK's Pet Travel Scheme was extended to the new 'Accession States', I couldn't visit these regions with my dog, and bring her back to the UK without her enduring six months of quarantine. Now, with her paperwork in order, I can take Macy with me as my travelling companion and I won't have to worry about putting her into quarantine when we return to the UK.

*　　*　　*

Although I was born, raised and educated in Canada, I've lived in Britain for so long that I've contracted through osmosis the British habit of looking upon the rest of Europe as a slightly curious place, semi-detached from Britain—great for holidays, but in all other aspects quite alien and strange. What is 'Europe'? What are its geographical limits? Where is its heart? Technically, the geographical heart of Europe is— strange as it sounds—a few kilometres north-west of Vilnius in Lithuania, but culturally, I still can't help but think that Europe ends somewhere around the eastern forests of Austria.

Of course, our governments tell us there's no

European heartland, that we're all Europeans, free to live and work anywhere within the European Union. Should I define 'Europe' as anywhere where I can freely work? I don't really know what 'Europe' is or what it means. Do you?

For most of my life, 'Europe' meant 'Western Europe', post-war capitalist Europe, from Norway and Sweden south through Denmark, Germany and Switzerland to Italy, and from Portugal, east through Spain and France and the Benelux countries to Germany. When I was young, Finland and Austria were almost European; they were associate countries that, by the time I was in my teens, had become part of 'my' Europe.

A century earlier, the definition of Europe was quite different. When Macy—my golden retriever—and I walk in Kensington Gardens in London we pass a sculpture of 'Europe' on the south-west corner of the Albert Memorial. Judging from this piece of nineteenth-century kitsch, the Victorians had an even more restricted definition of what the word meant: 'Europe' is represented by Britain, France, Germany and Italy alone.

The sculpture was unveiled in 1876, just five years after Bismarck unified Germany, but the principalities that made up Europe's newest nation-state had been falling in and out of alliance for centuries, first under the Holy Roman Empire and then under the German Confederation. 'Germany', even before it existed as the nation it now is, was the epicentre of the enduring friction between Europe's East and West. So is Germany the true heart of Europe?

The German language and German culture certainly dominated a vast, ever-changing region

6

that came to be known loosely as 'Mitteleuropa' which extended to the edges of the Black Sea and the Mediterranean in the south-east and south (under the Hapsburgs) and to Poland's present-day border with Belarus in the north-east (under Prussia). By the time of my grandparents' birth, merchants from Königsberg in East Prussia (now Russia's Kaliningrad) dominated business and culture further up the Baltic, as far north as the Gulf of Finland.

After World War Two, of course, the eastern parts of 'Mitteleuropa' fell under Soviet control, and the Russians set about eliminating all traces of German influence. For a generation, East and West were deadlocked in the Cold War. This is the region I'm most interested in visiting.

My father and his siblings never asked their parents about 'the old country'. Nor did my mother and her siblings, all born in or near Toronto, question their family. More often than not, those who left continental Europe in the late 1800s for a better life elsewhere were not just finding a new place to live, they were creating a whole new identity for themselves. It was a fresh start, a new beginning, a new country, new values and just as often a fresh, new name. Emigrants seldom looked back.

JR Fogle's and Leah Bernard's parents were products of 'Mitteleuropa'. Our family names may have been German—'Vogel' and 'Berhardt'—anglicised to 'Fogle' and 'Bernard' when they reached Britain.

The culture of Mitteleuropa had a remarkably strong assimilated Jewish element to it. The concept and culture of Mitteleuropa was virtually

7

destroyed during World War Two. What little survived went into hibernation as Germany turned in on itself and faced its past, and the eastern part of Mitteleuropa was vindictively brutalised by the Soviet Union's occupation. That most recent chapter in Europe's 1000-year civil war between West and East, between German and Russian lands, reached its latest truce in 1989 when it became possible once more for people on both sides of the Iron Curtain to travel with ease to each other's lands.

When I first visited Europe in 1964 at the height of the Cold War it was only really practical to travel in 'Western Europe', almost impossible—especially if you were driving, as I was—to visit Soviet-zone cities like Prague, Leipzig, Budapest or Warsaw. Since 1989 I've visited Budapest and Prague a couple of times but I haven't spent a single day in the countryside of any former Soviet country. Most Western Europeans who travel into old 'Mitteleuropa' stick to the cities.

What is the countryside, the former heartland of the continent, like? I don't know, but I want to find out.

*　　　*　　　*

Here in Sussex, where I am right now, it's spring. A collared dove, a species that didn't venture much farther north than Venice when I was a boy, is cooing down the chimney into the back of my consciousness. There was a fierce nor'easter last night, and an unexpected hoar-frost this morning that has coated the grass like snow. The lawn is covered by branches whipped from the walnut

8

tree, lying like shipwrecks on a frothy white sea.

Under a low, grey sky Macy and I went for our morning walk in the fields across the lane from my house. Creamy white yarrow as tall as I am lined the footpath through a pungent field of rape which was blindingly yellow even under the overcast sky. We passed a just-ploughed field on which at least 100 crows were resting. I saw a fox with mange so severe that it would probably eventually kill it, but Macy didn't spot it so she didn't give chase. She concentrated on the pheasants and grouse and rabbits.

A cuckoo, sounding like a slowed-down version of an old French police siren called from the distant, just-budding trees. The field by the railway line looked like a faded old Turkish rug, an inviting carpet of greens, browns and mauve, and everywhere the smell of crushed camomile, a weed of cultivation, filled the air as Macy raced through the fields picking up more animal scent. The first ox-eye daisies, already over half a metre high, had just opened and beneath them were countless egg-yolk yellow dandelions and paler yellow sow thistles. It was grey and dull and threatening and bleak, and I wore two coats because of the bite to the wind, and I loved it.

To me, the landscape is as exciting as the people who live in it. What you can grow on the land; what lives in it or on it; how the land's location and form affects the weather—all of these create the spirit of a place. Nature affects culture too, just as much as it determines the wildflowers or wildlife that inhabit a locale. Firm cultural evidence that the Baltic is the region where my family originated survived in my father's and, as a consequence, in

9

my own taste memories: a love of herring, especially when it's marinated with sweet onions in sour cream and served with a crunchy, dill pickle. Regional cultures bear the signature of the material with which nature provides them.

When Macy and I travel through the rural heartlands of the Great European Plain, I want to see for myself what the land is like and how people live on it and from it. I'm curious: are the consequences of the Soviet occupation still being felt? Has joining the EU made any difference? Why do young people from this region of the continent decamp in their hundreds of thousands to others' countries—especially the UK and Ireland—to work?

The Alpine mountain ranges that stretch from the Pyrenees by the Atlantic through the Swiss-Italian-Austrian Alps to the Polish-Slovakian Tatras and on to the Black Sea mark the natural physical division between Northern Europe and Southern Europe. My plan is to remain, until the latter part of the trip, north of this natural divide, travelling east from London across the unending flatlands of the Great European Plain that stretches 4000 kilometres from the Atlantic to Russia's Ural Mountains. There may be hills in northern Europe, here and there, but, say the geographers, Harrow-on-the-Hill in suburban west London is the highest point of land until you reach the Urals. Over that distance, the land falls 40 centimetres per kilometre, 26 inches per mile. That's a 0.04 per cent gradient.

The Great Plain is Northern Europe's dominant feature and historians argue that it was the lack of natural territorial limits, more than any other factor, that nourished Europe's interminable civil war. Visually, I imagine it's a bland, emotionless landscape, which is doubtless why this is the region of Europe least visited by tourists. Isolated in pockets throughout the Great Plain are ancient, urban concentrations, some of Europe's most historic cities—Kracow, Warsaw, Riga, Vilnius, L'viv, Kiev—but with a few exceptions I'll avoid cities and travel through rural lands.

The rivers I'll cross—the Meuse, Rhine, Weser, Elbe, Neiman, Necker and Vistula—all meander north over this gentle gradient to the North and Baltic Seas. Only near the end of my journey, when I crest the hills of south-east Poland and Slovakia will the watershed change and rivers flow to the Black Sea, the Adriatic or the Mediterranean. It strikes me that, just as there is a physical gradient across the Great European Plain, you can perceive a cultural gradient too. The westerly culture often looks down on the culture of the east. Consider the French attitude to the Belgians and Germans, the German attitude to the Poles and Slavs and the Pole's attitude to the Russians and Ukrainians. Or, for that matter, the Swedes' attitude to the Finns and the Russians' attitude to people from the Central Asian republics of their old Empire. The further east you live, it seems, the more 'primitive' you are. Conversely, eastern cultures are aspirational, yearning for the commercial or artistic and scientific success of their western neighbours.

I'm curious to see where my antecedents lived and, if possible, to find out more about how they lived. Julia, my wife, has an antique fair in London in the latter part of October where I can help so

11

I've only got 45 days before I have to be back. There's a lot of ground to cover in a short time so I'll be constantly moving on.

*   *   *

To guide me, I'm taking my collection of *Baedeker Guides* from the late 1800s and early 1900s, together with my battered copy of Eric Frommer's *Europe on $5 a Day*, my bible on my first visit to Europe in 1964, and also the diary I kept on that four-month trip. I've got modern road maps but will also have with me my 1964 leather-bound *Kummerly & Frey European Road Atlas* and, much more useful and exciting, the 1938 edition of *L'Europe en Automobile*, the official guide to driving through Europe published by the International Association of Automobile Clubs, with maps also by Kummerley & Frey.

Oh yes, and I'll have Sat Nav Barry, my disembodied Australian guide should be helpful. He even knows Poland. I'm also taking with me a bird book, a wildflower book, a trees and shrubs book, a wild herb book, a national parks of Europe book and Norman Davies's scintillating *Europe, a History*. You should read that book. It's superb.

My plan is for us to travel when kids across Europe have returned to school after their summer break, in September and October. I'll drive and live in a Roadtrek, a compact, extremely well-fitted Canadian-made motorhome. I'm importing a used one from Florida. 'Us' means Macy and me. Julia will remain at the other end of the phone at home, riding herd on our family and running her antiques business.

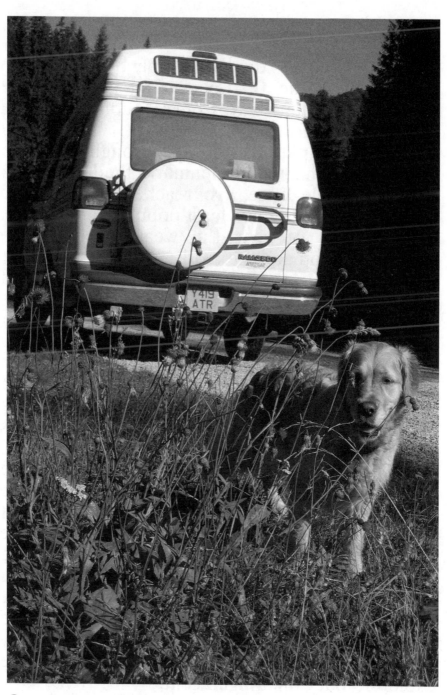

Our home away from home

*　　　*　　　*

Part of our route is dictated simply by the need to 'get there' in the first place and getting there means going a long way, from London to Finland before reaching Estonia, my first 'new' EU country. The plan is to nip through Holland, northern Germany and Denmark, then ease back on the throttle once I've reached Sweden and Finland, the continent's least populated countries. At this time of year the weather should be reasonably good and the roads should be deserted. It also gives me the opportunity to visit some of the remote Baltic islands that British tourists seldom visit: Sweden's Öland and Gotland, Finland's Åland and Estonia's Saaremaa.

*　　　*　　　*

For most of the year, Macy, my travel buddy, leads the life of a typical 'middle class' dog. We have a morning walk together in the park before I leave for work. Later in the day, either Julia or I take her for another 45 minutes of exercise and the rest of the time she's a couch potato. It's a shame because, of all the dogs I've lived with, Macy is the most 'dogged'. Indoors she's a bit dour, a serious dog, not much of a comedian, sensitive to the unexpected, tentative about life. Outdoors she transmogrifies into Macy the Fearless, Macy the Mischievous, Macy the Intrepid, Macy the Explorer, Macy the Magnificent.

I've travelled extensively with her before. We spent almost three months together journeying around North America in a spacious, vintage motorhome. On those travels I watched as she honed her hunting skills until she was capable of anticipating an animal's zigs and zags, and was even catching desert hares. When we returned to England she continued to use her skills. Her objective was to make Sussex a rabbit-free county. She has nearly succeeded, and our local farmer is very grateful.

Macy is NOT, however, a good driving companion. When I'm driving a motorhome, and she can freely walk around, she pesters. 'Are we there yet?' 'Can we stop soon?' 'Is it much farther?' 'Is there a less bumpy road?' 'If I pant like this, will you feel sorry for me and let me out?' She's a boring traveller, not a scenery hound. She never, ever looks out the window, but as soon as the engine is turned off you can almost feel the electricity surge through her body.

As the door opens, rain or shine, she throws herself outside, eats up the landscape with her eyes, ears and nose, then dances in anticipation as I climb out of the motorhome and choose the direction we walk in. She will walk, trot, canter or gallop for as long as I let her. Her inquisitiveness never flags. Her alertness never diminishes. She is a perfect hiking companion. Each walk is a master class in the art of observing nature.

Her nose is my best guide. Given what that nose has lead me to in the past, I'm sure it'll turn up plenty of surprises on our travels. Macy will be my social secretary too—she's fluently multilingual, superb at intuitively understanding all European languages. On the other hand I only understand English and a smattering of the Romance languages.

This should be fine until I leave Scandinavia but may be problematic in 'new' Europe, so I'm making a few contacts before leaving and combining the business of travelling with some professional pleasure. I wish I could explain to Mace right now that in a few months' time she'll get petted and pummelled to her heart's content when I'm in Vilnius, birthplace of my great-great-great-great-great-great-great-grandfather. I've just got an invitation to speak in the city at a meeting of the Golden Retriever Breeders' Club of Lithuania, and she's the guest of honour.

Bruce Fogle
London
April 2005

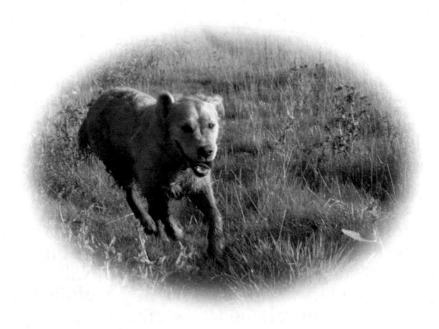

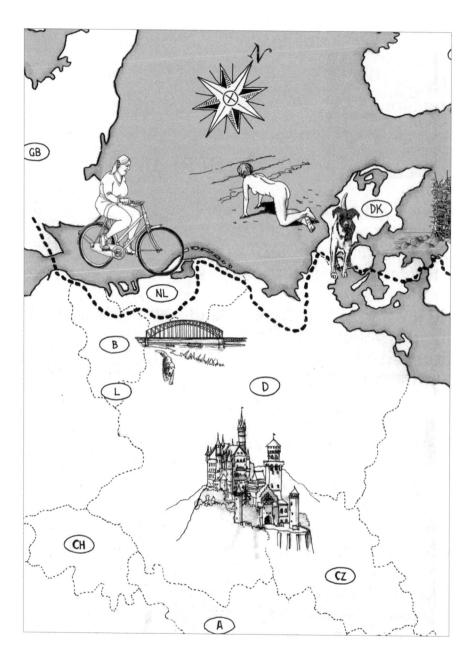

CHAPTER ONE

AROUND THE NORTH SEA

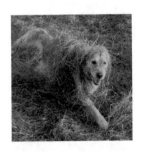

THE NETHERLANDS

People per square kilometre	*441*
Dogs per square kilometre	*42*
Average height of Dutch women	*5'8"*
Average height of British women	*5'4"*

Macy was in her element, and so was I. Enveloped by the deliciously sweet aroma of just-cut hay, we were exploring the banks of the Rhine near Arnhem in the Netherlands. The sun was about to set and although it was early September it was still hot, really hot—T-shirt and shorts weather. There's an ancient dike along the southern side of the river, but here on the northern bank is a flood plain extending over 500 metres to the rising elevations of the town of Oosterbeek.

Macy had found a ball and a blonde, and the leggy blonde was throwing the ball into a field of drying hay for Macy to retrieve. Macy would find the ball, somersault and roll in the fragrant hay, then return it to the blonde for another toss. The equally fragrant Dutch blonde would say 'Dish on veranda, hound,' or something that sounded like that, stroke Macy's head and toss the ball again. It was enchanting. Each time the blonde threw the ball, she threw it a little further, and now she wound up and lobbed a powerful overarm pitch to the far end of the field. The tennis ball sailed high into the sky, and so did her halter top. It settled on her gorgeous blonde head. I was really pleased to be in Holland.

An enchanting giggle and liberated breasts, what an unexpected way to start a road trip. We both grinned. Well, I sure did—I can't really tell with Macy. She's a bit bipolar, my dog. Indoors she may seem almost emotionless, a quiet, still dog. But when she's outdoors, in her natural element, she has a thrilling vibrancy about her, a confident, questing interest in anything her senses capture.

We'd left London earlier in the day in our small motorhome that had only just cleared Customs. Mace enjoys the consequences of travel, not travel itself. To make matters worse for her, the Roadtrek had a typical 'soft' American suspension, and tipped into curves, constantly rolling her out of her bed. I'd set Barry the Sat Nav for Arnhem and obediently went where my Australian navigator directed me. We stopped a couple of times in Belgium, once for Macy to have a break in a field of drying rapeseed, and again by a field of sweetcorn where she amused herself by tearing after a hare across the stubble of a cut wheatfield while I borrowed a couple of cobs of corn for dinner.

Holland started to grow on me when I overruled Barry, left the charmless motorway and took the old oak-lined road to 's-Hertogenbosch. This was how I remembered the Netherlands from my first visit here over 40 years ago, the neat little homes with clean, curtainless windows, well-groomed, topiaried gardens, fastidiously trimmed verges, symmetrically cut fields and well dressed people on orderly bicycle paths languorously pedalling their old-fashioned 'sit up and beg' bikes.

At Heteren my road map showed a secondary road paralleling the Rhine so I headed for what turned out to be a scary, very narrow strip of tarmac running along the top of a precipitous dike on the south bank of the Rhine. Fruit farms flanked the southern side of the dike and I stopped at one, buying pears from a young farmer. It may sound easy but it took fearsome bravery on my part to negotiate the steep 8-metre decline off the dike to the farmhouse far below, though the climb back up to the road was dead easy. My new home had unexpectedly immense power. That was reassuring.

In Oosterbeek, just outside Arnhem, as evening was approaching I saw a faded camping sign pointing down toward the Rhine and took the road through old suburbs of tightly packed houses, eventually emerging on to a dirt road through open fields that dead-ended in a grove of trees at 'Camping/Jachthaven Oosterbeeks Rijnoever'. What an unexpected treat—only minutes away from the congested roads of Oosterbeek, I'd found a virtually empty campsite, surrounded by pastureland, where I could park for the night on grass less than 10 metres from a sandy beach on the banks of the Rhine.

I fed Macy and we went to scout out the surroundings. Tundra swans glided silently along the river, unperturbed by a powerboat taking a wet-suit clad water skier for a final few spins. Further out in the river a long, low, black barge churned towards Rotterdam while to the east, towards Arnhem, trains clicked over a cantilevered rail bridge—the one that had been the focus of the war film *A Bridge Too Far*.

After beachcombing, and being welcomed by the ball-throwing blonde in such an accommodating way, Macy and I walked along 'Polderweg' the dead-end dirt road leading to the campsite, in the still, warm evening. Songbirds in the pollarded willows by the road serenaded a lean, lone man who was cutting hay with a scythe. Macy trotted obediently along beside me, occasionally darting into the verge to follow scents or sounds, through flowering nettle, buttercups, toadflax and ox-eye daisies—'marguerites' here in continental Europe.

White flowering bindweed wrapped itself around fence posts, trees, even grasses and weeds, giving a peaceful unity to our surroundings. Above the bindweed, heavy masses of deep purple elderberries drooped from the ends of branches and crimson rosehips glistened in the last rays of the sun. All around us was the uplifting, intoxicating smell of the drying hay. Three shaggy ponies grazing in an adjacent field came over for a tickle and as they did so, in the pink light of sunset a flock of starlings rose and fell in magical synchrony. It was all so unexpected, so unforeseen, so un-Dutch in densely populated Holland.

I inaugurated the Roadtrek's kitchen that night by boiling my fresh-picked Belgian sweetcorn then dicing the local pears to mix with blackberries just picked from the Polderweg verge. Macy had a Krispy Kreme donut. I'd brought a dozen for her to have as special treats on boring days. I fell asleep relaxed and easy on that first night of our journey, to the sound of a screeching owl, trains traversing the Arnhem bridge, barges chugging towards Rotterdam and images of blondes playing ball with dogs.

I'd forgotten how perfectly at home I always feel in Holland. I like the people and that's a vestige of both my childhood and my Canadian nationality. When I was a little boy in Toronto, all the growers who delivered to my father's flower-shop were Dutch and whenever I went to visit him at work these rough-handed giants would ritually lift me in the air as a manly 'hello', before filling my father's green tin containers with water to stand the cut flowers in. I enjoyed that; it's an indelible memory.

I enjoyed the company of my favourite uncle too, a Dutchman, Bram, born north of Amsterdam, in Alekmaar, where cheese auctions historically took place. He was a diamond polisher by trade, a trout fisherman by inclination—an immigrant to Canada in 1940 who had married my father's sister. I admired Holland too, a virtual man-made land. Polderisation—the creation of habitable land from shallows or marshland—started in the 1200s and still continues. I appreciate Dutch tolerance, Dutch thrift, the Dutch work ethic. For me, the Dutch—at least once upon a time—were honest and industrious and Holland was filled with little boys who saved countries by sticking their fingers in leaking dikes.

When I first visited the Netherlands in 1964 it was less than 25 years since Germany had invaded the neutral Netherlands and the Dutch Royal Family had escaped to London. As Britain faced invasion, Queen Wilhelmina arranged for her daughter Princess Juliana, together with Juliana's husband Prince Bernhard and their two children,

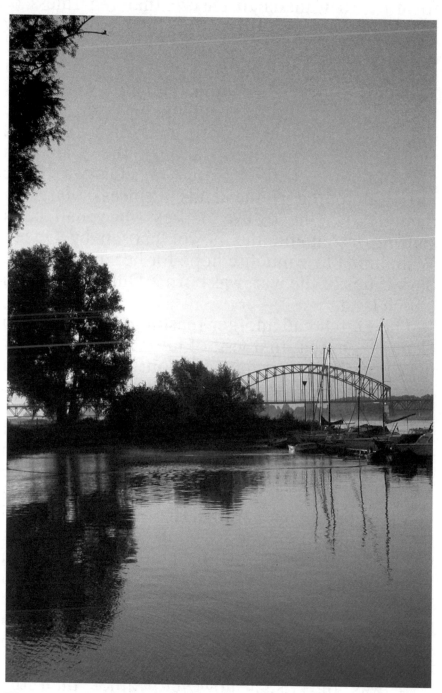

THE CANTILEVERED RAIL BRIDGE AT ARNHEM

to move to Canada to ensure that regardless of what happened in Europe, the Dutch Royal Family would survive.

While living in Canada, in the Ottawa suburb of Rockcliffe, near Britannia Heights where my father grew up, Princess Juliana gave birth to the only royal baby ever born in North America. Before she went into labour, the Canadian government ceded a room at Ottawa Civic Hospital to the Netherlands. Princess Margriet, named after the ox-eye daisies Macy had been sniffing last night, the flower chosen by Queen Wilhelmina to symbolise hope for her nation in the dark times of the war, was born a Dutch citizen on Dutch land.

The Dutch had another reason to be grateful to Canada. On that first visit of mine in 1964, I never once paid for accommodation: my Canadian passport was a ticket into Dutch homes. I was given rooms to sleep in and meals to eat, and I was taken to war cemeteries. 'Was your father here?' I was relentlessly asked. It was Canadian troops who liberated Belgium and the Netherlands from the Germans. The commander of the occupying German forces, General Blaskowitz, surrendered to Lieutenant-General Foulkes of the 1st Canadian Army Corps. In gratitude, a million tulips bloom in Ottawa every spring as a gift from the Dutch Royal Family, and are refreshed each year by an annual gift of 20,000 more. As the son of a florist, how can I possibly not like a nation that 'says it with flowers'?

It was the visual however, rather than the historical, that induced me to bide my time and stay longer in Holland; the unexpected sight of

Sahara-like sand dunes, of a cork-dry desert landscape in the heart of the country. In my 1888 edition of *Baedeker's Belgium and Holland*, the fertile land by the Rhine where I camped was called the Betuwe or 'good island'. The sandy tract to the north, between Arnhem and the Zuiderzee, was called the Veluwe or 'barren island'. That sandy tract is now the Netherlands' largest National Park, De Hoge Veluwe, 'the high barren island' and this is where the sand dunes are located.

The roads in De Hoge Veluwe were empty of traffic. I parked and, sitting in warm sunshine amongst the purple heather, had breakfast while large white butterflies flitted around Macy who sat quietly, raising her head, closing her eyes, sniffing the air.

After breakfast, Macy and I walked alone through the purple sea, past occasional islands of oak and beech and majestic stands of Scots pines. As we walked, two sturdy Dutch girls in red-checked shirts, jeans and straw cowgirl hats, galloped past. They're really big, these Dutch girls. Or the horses are very small.

It was when we circled back to the Roadtrek that we came across the stark landscape of undulating hills of golden sand, wandering sand dunes tens of metres high and firm enough for climbing on.

This was an accidental landscape. Centuries ago, the covering trees in this region were cut for building or burning. Then the land was grazed to exhaustion. The remaining soil was stripped and mixed with sheep manure to make land elsewhere in Holland more fertile for growing crops.

Eventually what little soil remained was blown away, revealing the underlying ice-age, golden sand on which the heather now grew.

I followed Macy who raced gleefully up the dunes and entertained her by throwing bleached sticks for her to retrieve. At my feet were sand lizard tracks and around the occasional, sun-bleached, stump of a tree killed off long ago by the shifting sands, were miniscule mouse footprints. Here and there amongst the dunes were isolated trees, still somehow alive in the sand that was enveloping them. We sat, or at least I did, and soaked up the sun. Macy scent-trailed after rodents.

At the park's visitors' centre, I bought some locally produced 'koolzaad' honey, a smooth, tawny honey with an almost buttery taste, collected by bees from rape when it first flowers, and a cycling map, then mounted one of the 1700 bicycles available free to park visitors and pedalled out of the parking lot, Macy trotting obediently behind.

'What a well-trained dog you have,' an Amazon of a blonde Dutch woman said to me. I nodded in agreement.

'What a well-trained dog you have!' she shouted louder. I waved back.

'What a well-trained dog you have!' she screamed in admiration, but then I thought that maybe that wasn't what she was saying in Dutch, so I turned the bike around and pedalled back to her.

'I'm sorry I don't understand Dutch,' I explained as I tilted my head back 45° and looked up into her eyes.

'If you don't put your dog on a lead immediately

I will get my husband!' she thundered.

'Her husband?' I thought, 'Godzilla is 30 years younger than I am and could flatten me with a single pinkie. She needs her husband?'

'Not tough enough yourself, huh? Need your husband to back you up do you?' Macy challenged, giving the Amazon an unblinking stare, but I snapped the lead on to her collar and meekly bicycled away, yanking her along behind. The deciduous woodlands were open and bright but the coniferous woods were darker. There were woodlarks everywhere.

Deep in a conifer stand I stopped when I heard tapping from somewhere in the pine trees. Almost immediately above me I saw what looked like a crow with a pointed tail jackhammering the tree. I couldn't see the crown of its head but it had to be a black woodpecker. I'd never seen one before. At the northern end of the park, near the hunting lodge, we wandered past a lichen-clad headstone on which was engraved 'Schurftel'. I thought it must be a memorial to an itchy dog, but was told when I returned later to the visitors' centre that 'Schurftel', in Dutch means 'Scruffy', not 'Scurfy'. Scruffy had belonged to the family who donated De Hoge Veluwe to the nation. I wonder if he enjoyed the dunes as much as Macy did.

At the park campground that evening, a handsome couple in their seventies came to admire the Roadtrek. They had a caravan nearby and a season-pass to the park.

'It's never busy, even at the height of summer,' the man explained, as I took them both on a tour of the innards of my camper. I told him the vehicle was Canadian, as I was, and he replied, 'You know, we were liberated by Canadians. I lived 10 kilometres south of Groningen. When they came through we stood by our front gates, waving and saluting. My mother pushed apples and pears into their rucksacks. I don't know where she hid them from us. There was little food that winter.' I asked if he knew who the troops were, what parts of Canada they came from.

'It was the 2nd Canadian Infantry Division that liberated us. I remember exactly the names of your regiments. The Royal Hamilton Light Infantry. The Queen's Own Cameron Highlanders of Canada. The Toronto Scottish. Fort Garry Horse. The Canadian Hussars. The Black Watch of Canada. The Calgary Highlanders. The Maisonneuve Regiment. The Mont Royal Fusiliers. I particularly enjoyed the South Saskatchewan Regiment. What a wonderful word, "Saskatchewan". A wonderful word.' Without my further prompting and with his wife intently listening, he continued.

'It always fascinated me that Canadians and Australians and New Zealanders came from so far away to fight in Europe's wars. It disturbs me how the British used these troops. At Dieppe, at Monte Cassino, they were used as shock troops, as gun fodder. The Poles were used in the same fashion. I do not like that aspect. After the war many Polish troops could not go back home. Many found work in the mines here in Holland. We did not treat these people as we should have.'

When asked where I was going, I explained my route through the new countries of the European Union and mentioned that our governments— both mine and his—routinely remind us we're all

'Europeans'. He and his wife chuckled.

'I was 14 when the war ended,' he said. 'Today my children go to visit friends in Germany and my wife and I keep our mouths closed. We should not relive the past but I still cannot visit Germany.'

'After 50 years,' his wife added, 'it is only now becoming possible to talk about the war.'

GERMANY

People per square kilometre	*230*
Dogs per square kilometre	*14*
Nude pensioners per 100 metres on Sylt beaches	*14*

I don't know what to make of Germany. The Dutch couple, with memories of the war, can't forget what Germany did to the Netherlands yet have the moral strength not to infect their children with hatred. My image of modern Germany and Germans is vague. They're 'good Europeans' but I haven't got a firm idea what a modern 'German' is, unless that's exactly what a modern German is—*a good European*'. I wasn't going to find out on this trip though because we were only passing through quickly, with a brief detour off shore. Macy doesn't swim. She loves water—lying in it, wading in it, splashing in it, keeping her head under for over 30 seconds, searching in it for items to retrieve—but she doesn't swim. Now we were approaching wading-dog heaven. From the Dutch island of Texel (north of Alekmaar where my Uncle Bram was born), across the German frontier to the island of Sylt by the Danish border and then

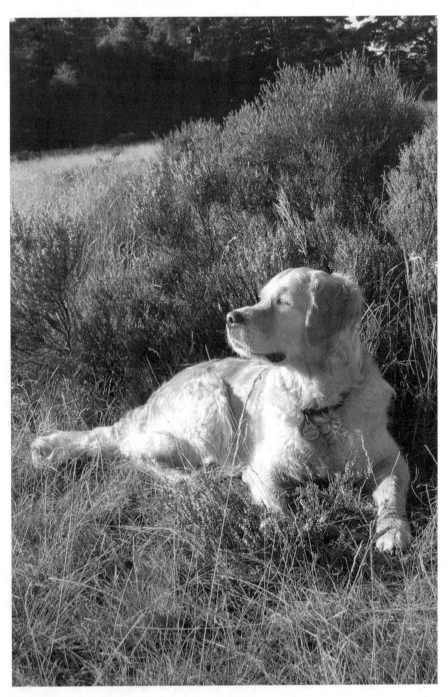

MACY SAT AND SOAKED UP THE SUN

to Rømø and Blavands Huk north of Esbjerg in Denmark lie the most extensive tidal-flats in the world.

This is where Europe's largest but perhaps least-known national park is, the Wadden Sea National Park. Wadden means 'shallow' in Dutch but the Wadden Sea is more than just that—it contains thousands of square kilometres of silty mud-flats, coarser sand-flats, sand-bars, marshes and low-lying islands. Some of these islands, the *'Halligen'* or 'un-diked islands' off the coast of German North Friesland, where we now were, are so low that they're completely inundated by frequent storm tides powering in from the North Sea. When that happens, only the island homesteads built high on artificial earthworks are visible above the surrounding, tormenting sea. This is one of the most environmentally turbulent regions of Europe.

We drove around the German Bight or Deutsche Bucht, listening to truly dire German Euro-pop. God it's awful, and it was on every single radio station. I stopped at a rest area where Macy disappeared into the bushes and when I followed I found her sniffing piles of human turds and tissues. On a tree was posted a sign, 'Welcome to environmentally conscious Germany where we recycle everything.' OK, there was no sign, but the turds were real. Mace told me they were all guy turds.

It's hard to escape war history in this region of Europe. It's a constant subtext. As I drove over the Kiel Canal towards Denmark, a convoy of container ships slowly passed beneath me. My marbled, gilt-stamped 1925 edition of *Baedeker's*

31

Northern Germany dryly states that, 'In accordance with the Treaty of Versailles the canal has been internationalised.' This was to prevent Germany from using it to move its fleet again, which was, after all, the main reason it was built the first place. In 1936 Hitler repudiated the canal's international status and restricted its use to German interests. Today it's once more the short-cut around Denmark for Baltic shipping.

This is the core of Schleswig-Holstein, a province that has yo-yoed between Germany and Denmark. In 1864, when it was part of Denmark, Prussia and Austria went to war with the Danes and quickly grabbed it. The Prussians got Schleswig while, curiously, the Austrians administered Holstein long-distance. That didn't last long. When the Austrians and Prussians warred with each other two years later, the whole of Schleswig-Holstein was incorporated into Prussia, which was soon to become the dominant state in a united Germany.

'We shall go out and bomb every building in Britain marked with three stars in the *Baedeker Guide,*' declared the Nazi propagandist Baron Gustav Braun Von Sturm after the RAF's misguided assault on the scenic but strategically unimportant German Baltic port of Lubeck. For over 100 years Baedeker guides were the acme of accuracy. Karl Baedeker began publishing his scrupulously researched urbane travel guides in the 1820s, and their popularity made them a cultural reference point in themselves. Lucy Honeychurch and her aunt Charlotte Bartlett tote their *Baedeker's Italy* everywhere in E M Forster's *A Room with a View*. In *A Tramp Abroad*, Mark

Twain quibbles, tongue in cheek, with Baedeker's factual accuracy. Baedeker states it takes three and a half hours to reach a peak above Lucerne while Twain said it took him three days.

Karl Baedeker's ambition was to provide readers with accurate, crystal-clear travel, hotel and cultural information, allowing them to dispense with paid human guides, who might be unreliable. He created the concept of the travel Bible, and the company he set up still publishes and updates travel guides. I used their modern and very boring *Baedeker's Autoguides* when I first visited Europe in 1964. Compared to their late-nineteenth and early-twentieth century ancestors, the modern guides have had personality bypasses—the old editions give a superb insight into cultural history, as well as straightforward touring information.

*   *   *

There are two ways to get to the German island of Sylt: by car train over a causeway from Germany, or by ferry from the Danish island of Rømø. I chose the latter. On a fresh, breezy, bright and clear morning I joined hundreds of big Germans in their big black cars on the 45 minute ferry journey to List at the north end of the island. This was fun for Macy as it seemed that most of my fellow grey-haired travellers had dogs with them, golden retrievers, spaniels, shih-tzus, spitzes, Newfoundlands and of course German shepherds. My dog enjoyed a considerable amount of head stroking and got to sniff quite a few new canine backsides on that trip, taking her mind off the fact that she doesn't like ferry crossings.

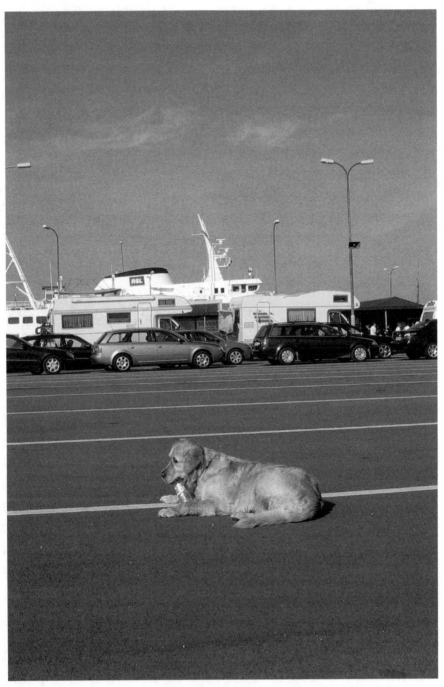

Rømø: waiting for the car ferry to Sylt

Sylt is quirky and it's rarely visited by the British, which is a shame because it's got great seashores and surprising shopping. It's enduringly popular with German tourists, though. Thomas Mann came and stayed; Theodor Storm wrote his *Sylt Novella* about the island; Stefan Zweig visited too, writing of his 'week of love in this mild wilderness' and it's easy to see what inspired him.

Sylt is a naturalist's paradise. We spent a day walking barefoot on the eastern edge of the island, sometimes on the firm salt-flats and sometimes through ankle-deep sludge, past shallow water filled with silt-grass and grasswort. Macy is, of course, always barefoot. I found that my boots were getting sucked into the sludge so I joined her.

Wading birds worked the mud-flats searching for worms, snails, mussels or simply feeding off the plankton and mats of algae covering the sediment. In the still water beyond the mud-flats thousands of brent geese sat motionless on the water. This is a tranquil landscape, relaxing, meditative, soothing, and the mother lode of one of Europe's most fertile ecosystems. At this time of year, a thimble of water on the eastern side of Sylt contains perhaps a million single cell micro-organisms. Tens of thousands of worms, snails and mini-crabs live in each square metre of silt. The Wadden Sea is the nursery for the North Sea's herring, sole and plaice. It's the most vital stopover for the millions of birds that migrate via the east Atlantic flyway each year, and feast on the fry. Seals and porpoises raise their young there too, plundering the rich supply of young fish.

A road runs down the spine of Sylt connecting List in the north to Hornum in the south, through heather heathland on which I saw clusters of rectangular, green-painted beehives. Dotted in the purple heath and amber dunes were groups of thatched villas, each surrounded by its own protective dike, so high that only the top half of each home was visible above them. Wooden steps over the dikes allowed access to the homes. The heather moorland climbed into low hills and valleys where we walked for hours alone. The inland was devoid of visitors. Those who were visiting were either in the towns or on the beaches that line the western side of the island.

*   *   *

Each year the power of the sea chews off a metre of these western beaches. In spring, massive pumps funnel a million cubic metres of sand back from the sea floor on to the shore. Although it was gusty, it was a warm wind that blew as we reached the heights of the dunes. Macy was in heaven, leaping through the dunes that rolled like verdant carpets to the brilliant white sandy beach and the startlingly azure sea beyond. A red-and-black hand-painted sign pointed towards the 'hundestrand'—the dog beach—200 metres to the right and I decided to walk there via the beach itself rather than the dunes.

There were walkers on the pristine sloping beach and I joined them while Macy ploughed through the pounding surf checking for flotsam, and found a red-and-white striped cork float which she proudly brought back to me. I took it from her and she marched ahead, tail high, sniffing razor clam shells in the sand and surf. Then a naked guy, older than I am, came swinging towards me. And then another. And another. I looked ahead and there was another old naked man ahead of me, walking in the same direction I was walking in, only slower. Macy was catching up to him and as she did so her nose arced up from the sand and her tail went high. 'No sniffing!' I shouted, but it was too late.

There were clothed people walking the beach too; I met an attractive woman walking a Hovawart—a German guarding breed that looks like a golden retriever, only leggier and larger—but there was a surprisingly large number of naked people, all walking close to the water. To avoid the risk of further cold noses up German bums we moved closer to the reeds that marked the onset of the dunes. There were odd pink objects every five metres or so in a line in front of the reeds and I couldn't make out what they were until I realised they were knees-up *hausfraus*, sunning parts of their bodies that the sun seldom reaches. It was like a wet lab at a gynaecologists' convention, not a good sight. Not at all.

The main town on Sylt, Westerland, is absolutely dreadful. The chunky, concrete high-rises may be luxurious but they are intrusive and unfriendly on such a flat sand-bar of an island. They destroy the low key ambience of the place. I wanted to tell the Harley Davison rider I saw in Westerland that wearing a World War Two German helmet may be cool in California but it's a bit wince-inducing in Germany but I didn't. Near the village of Kampen we climbed the island's highest dune and in the crystal light I could see the outlines of the German islands of Fohr and

Amrum to the south and Danish Rømø to the north. Wind farms lined the Danish coastline to the east. A wind-farm plantation is planned for the sea west of Sylt and I wondered how it will affect local wildlife.

The village of Kampen itself was filled with thatched luxury boutiques and terraced restaurants. Escada, Swarovski, Dolce & Gabbana, Jil Sander, Louis Vuitton, Hermès, Bulgari, Cartier—it was bizarre to find myself on a Bond Street, a 5th Avenue, a Rodeo Drive, in the middle of mud-flats and nothingness. Most of the shops had water bowls for dogs outside their doors and at one, a clothing shop, Macy was offered water and a hug and invited inside to share the shop assistant's food.

In Kampen, I met Dieter, a Hamburg snow remover, at a terraced restaurant where I stopped for a seafood salad. He spends the summer and autumn on Sylt. His 12-year-old Siberian husky who tried to attack each small dog that walked past, wore a kerchief on his neck. Dieter wore a cravat.

'Millions of people now visit Sylt,' he told me, 'especially on weekends because that is when train tickets are cheap. It's like Venice. We want tourists here but the right type of tourists. So now there is a tax just to visit a beach. The wicker beach-chairs, they are very Sylt. You can buy them in town but most weekend visitors only buy a Sylt sticker for their car to show off that they have visited.'

I'd seen the stickers, like drippy ink blobs the shape of the island, on the bumpers of so many of those big black cars. With a stranger to talk to, Dieter decided to tell me about 'the Germans'.

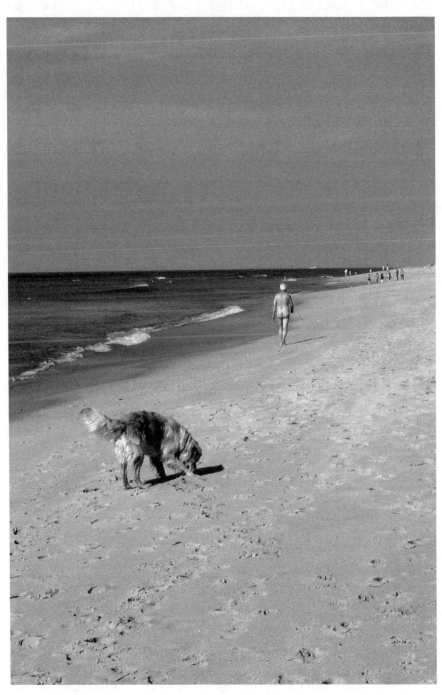

ENCOUNTERS WITH THE BEACH BUMS OF SYLT

'The Germans have a strange love/hate relationship with the British. They hate you for not being part of Europe and at the same time they envy you for not being part of Europe. You British, you do little things badly. The Germans, they do big things badly. World War One. World War Two. Of course 1989 is not in the same category but they have done it just as badly.' Dieter used 'they', not 'we' when he talked about the Germans. By '1989', he meant, of course, the reunification of East and West Germany.

'It was impetuous. Thoughtless. The Bundesbank said the Ostmark should not be exchanged for the Deutschmark but the politicians did not listen. You know, the East German government was a Nazi government. It was no better than Hitler. My stepsister is from East Germany. I used to visit her often but since 1989 I've never been back. You know why? Because the East is a piece of shit. It's not their fault that they expect the government to do everything for them. That's how they were educated. But it's a piece of shit. It will take another generation, before they understand you need to made decisions yourself. Work hard. Have goals.'

Dieter didn't think much of German industry either.

'Grundig, Blaupunkt, Mercedes, Siemens, they were the best. Now they are shit. Only Porsche continues to understand quality,' and he pointed to a silver Porsche parked directly in front of the restaurant.

'Do you know what the "HH" signifies on my auto licence? "Hansestadt Hamburg". The Hanseatic City of Hamburg. The Germans still live in the past, as if the Hanseatic League will rise again and they will dominate trade once more.'

I asked him where he learned his excellent English and he explained that after World War Two, his mother went to England where she washed hair for a living. She made friends and he continues to visit Devon regularly. 'One of my uncles was a prisoner of war in Canada. When the war ended and the Canadians arranged for him to return here, he asked to stay. Many did, and the Canadians were welcoming. Until he died two years ago I also visited him in Guelph, Ontario. He was a janitor at the university.'

The same university where I spent eight years at veterinary school.

DENMARK

People per square kilometre	*123*
Dogs per square kilometre	*14*
Truly Great Danes	*Niels Bohr, Søren Kierkegaard, Hans Christian Andersen, but not the 'Great Dane'*

'Jeg søger efter markedet,' he shouted from across the park. 'I'll have my coffee black, thanks,' I crisply replied, after quickly checking out what he'd asked me, according in my infallible, all-in-one pocket translation guide to all Europe's languages.

'Ah, you are English! We don't see many English here. There is supposed to be a farmers'-market somewhere in the park today.'

41

I was in Sønderborg, at the bottom of Danish Jutland, by the German border, staying in an asphalted campground—really a parking lot—by a wood overlooking the yacht harbour. My 1925 *Baedeker's Northern Germany* had advice on what I should see in Sønderburg even though it had been returned to Danish rule when the Danish-German border was redefined after World War One, five years before the book was published. A minute's walk from where I camped was the Sønderborg Bugt, or Sønderborg Bight, and that's where Macy and I were taking an early morning walk through the extensive parkland that abuts the shore.

'I'm surprised,' I replied to the man. 'It's so beautiful here, I'd expect you'd get lots of tourists.'

'Indeed we do,' he responded in immaculate English. 'We have the good fortune to be Germany's small neighbour.'

The wryness of his reply wasn't lost on me. I'd only met a few people in the countries bordering Germany but, 60 years after World War Two, it was still on their minds.

The sunshine was glorious. After leaving Sylt I found I didn't want to leave the coast yet, and neither did Macy, who loved walking the sun-washed beaches and snuffing up the sea air as much as I did, so we spent a day on the Danish island of Rømø.

Four times wider than Sylt, and, as a result, able to sustain agriculture, it is still only six kilometres from east to west. After walking through vistas of flowering sea roses, lyme and marram grasses, it was still over a kilometre from the onset of the sandy beach on the west side of the island to the water's edge.

That fresh sea air! Is there anything as invigorating? Further south the expansive sandy beach was even broader, at least three kilometres wide. The flat sands at Sønderstrand looked like Daytona Beach on racing day as dozens of Danes raced their cars to near the water to put in a day of wind surfing or, more envy-making, sand-sailing. I asked a sand sailer how far in the tides came before deciding exactly where to camp that evening.

*   *   *

At the fishing port of Havneby I saw my first ever *'Dansk-Svensk Gaardhund'* or Danish-Swedish Farmdog. One of my 'professional' objectives on this trip was to see, in the flesh, breeds of Scandinavian and Eastern European dogs that are extremely rare in Britain, or are not even represented there. Unexpectedly, here in the harbour, tied at the end of a red rope was a handsome, shiny tricolour specimen with a black-and-tan triangular head on a black-and-white body. I'd written about the breed before, but never actually seen one. They're just too uncommon. Before leaving London I'd arranged to meet another uncommon Danish dog breed, the Broholmer, but failed to find a breeder of the even rarer *Dansk-Svensk Gaardhund*, with its curiously political name.

Like farmers everywhere, Danes have always kept versatile dogs to rat and mouse, to herd cows into the milking parlour, to stand watch over the home or simply for the kids to play with. These short haired, 10 kilogram, pinscher-type dogs were

43

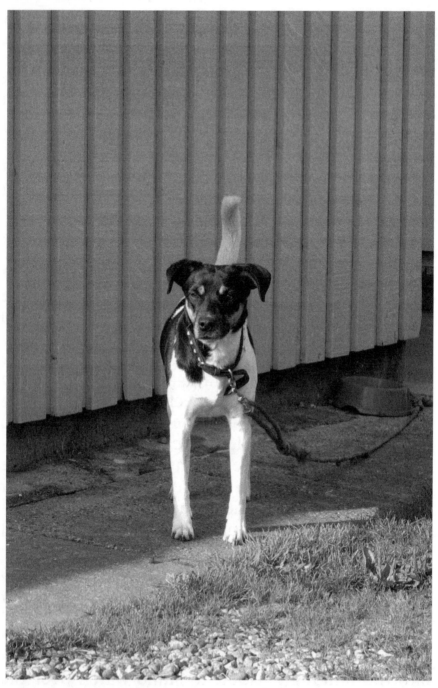

MY FIRST EVER 'DANSK-SVENSK GAARDHUND' OR
DANISH-SWEDISH FARMDOG

common not only in Denmark but also in neighbouring Schleswig-Holstein and in the southern Swedish province of Skåne across the Øresund strait from Copenhagen, a region that was once part of Denmark.

Fifty years ago, local farmers called them 'rat dogs' but as small farms disappeared so too did their rat dogs. City folk wanted dachshunds, not rural mutts. When the rat dog was on the verge of extinction however, it was rescued by dog breeders. They mated surviving examples of the dog in Sweden and Denmark (hence the name), but now also bred for a very unterrier-like affability, lack of aggression, and equable temperament. The dog I was now saying *'Godmorgen'* to was created as a result of this effort. I asked around and was told he was a fishing boat dog that went to sea with his master.

A 10 kilometre causeway over still, shallow water and salty marshland took us from Rømø back to the Jutland peninsula where hundreds of sheep grazed the salt-marsh. The coastal land is spatula-flat, protected from storm tides by an impressively high dike, a sea wall over a kilometre in from the sea. I walked westerly over the rise of the dike, and saw a seemingly endless grassland then marshland beyond it, the sea far in the distance. Winter storms will roll right in, sometimes surging the water right up to the dike itself. According to the girls tending the graveyard at Vesterend Ballum church when I visited, the dike was breached and the entire region flooded in January 1976. Only the church remained above water.

Farmers were busy. Combine harvesters worked

some fields while ploughs churned over the soil in others, inevitably followed by hundreds of opportunist gulls. The smell of damp fields being ploughed was earthy and comforting. The sky remained a perfect blue and the days warm, although the nights were now cooler. In Bredebrø I bought red peppers and dill from a roadside stand with an honour box for payment, and three types of herring—*'sild'*—from the local supermarket. On my way to Sønderborg I picked some ripe red apples from a tree growing on a rural verge and bought a bag of Danish new potatoes which I washed clean in the Sønderborg Bight.

*   *   *

I was still getting used to my home-away-from-home and in Sønderborg I rearranged my bedding. Until now I'd slept in a single bed. I'd planned to use the matching bunk as a sofa but I hadn't sat on it once. Each evening, after making dinner, I'd swivel the front passenger seat around, drop down the arm rests, sit and eat facing into the 'living-room'. I found I preferred to put my plate on my lap rather than put the table up. The passenger 'captain's chair' was also perfect for sitting in while I downloaded pictures into my computer and for transcribing notes from my little lighter-size digital recorder. Macy had taken to sleeping in the West Wing, up front on the floor by the kitchen and front seats, so it was no loss to her when I converted the back of the camper into a queen-size bed.

Macy didn't enjoy the 50-minute crossing over

the Lille Bælt from Jutland to Funen, in a bucking bronco of a ferry, so we stopped in quaint Fabørg to recover and have a coffee and, of course, a Danish. I didn't order any for her but the sight of a calm golden retriever sitting at a table outside a *konditori* on a cobbled street brings out a natural nurturing instinct in 18 to 25-year-old women. They swooped on Macy.

Listening to these girls ask Macy if she wanted some of their croissants reminded me how odd spoken Danish sounds. Lilting, tonal Swedish is one of the most beautiful of all European languages to listen to, but Danish sounds like Cockney spoken through a mouthful of ball bearings; syllables get swallowed or disappear completely. When my dog feeders realised I was English they launched into motherese in perfect American-English, in tone and words that Macy fully understood.

We lingered not. Having recuperated after the trauma of the rough crossing, we took the scenic southern route around Funen to the majestic Størebælt suspension bridge through a rolling landscape dotted with farms, past fields of wheat and corn waiting to be harvested, fields that had just been harvested and fields that were now being tilled. I stopped at another roadside honour stand where, with dragonflies hovering to check that I was honest, I bought a jar of tawny-coloured set honey as smooth and subtle as the De Hoge Veluwe Dutch rape flower honey.

*   *   *

We drove on through intermittent beech and oak

woodlands, past mature majestic chestnuts and maples, along rows of poplars and hazels and always, by the roadside, marguerites. This was an unexpectedly relaxing journey. Funen is bucolic, pastoral, idyllic in September in a way that reminded me of rural Sussex and Hampshire.

POTATO, APPLE AND HERRING SALAD
Peel and boil just-dug Danish new potatoes, dice them, cover them in olive oil and let them cool.
Unroll local Danish herring marinated with sugar and onions and cut each fillet into two-centimetre sections.
Core just-picked Danish red apples and cut them into thin wedges, leaving the skins on.
Combine everything and add a few squirts of balsamic vinegar.
Sprinkle with some pungent, fresh picked, chopped dill.
Sit in warm sunshine, with tortoiseshell butterflies flitting by, with a dog rolling on her back and kicking her legs in the air amongst golden wheat stubble, in a field of gently rolling hills in Funen. Eat your lunch.

From the bridge over the Størebælt across Zealand to Copenhagen then north to Elsinore and Hørnbæk I stuck to motorways, a decision Macy thoroughly approved of. I enjoy Copenhagen and would have stopped for a couple of days if I didn't have my dog with me. In 1964 I wrote a supplemental calculus exam here.

While travelling on my four-month visit to Europe that year, I learned that I had failed that subject in my spring exams but managed—I can't remember how—to arrange the rewrite here in Denmark rather than return to Canada. The accommodation bureau at the train station found me a home to live in for 10 days with a Jewish family who were amongst the 7000 who, over several nights in 1943, were smuggled by their fellow Danes, under the very noses of the Germans across the Øresund to neutral Sweden, where they remained until the end of the war.

The Germans managed to kill less than 100 Danish Jews, compared to over 100,000 Dutch ones. When the Danes returned to their homes in 1945 they saw that in their absence their gardens had been tended, their pets cared for and their possessions left intact.

*   *   *

North of Elsinore I stopped for a walk in a dense, silver-trunked, beech wood where plantations of mushrooms grew from old rotting tree stumps. Barry, my Australian Sat Nav man brought me to the Andersen's front door, a mean feat as they lived, as best a Dane can, in the middle of nowhere. I'd made contact with the Andersen family through Charlotte, a young family friend of theirs, who ran a website about Broholmer dogs, and they had invited me to meet their pack.

I visit Scandinavia frequently and feel as at ease here as I do in the Netherlands. I admire their ideal of what family life should be: snug, warm, cosy, intimate, free from stress or trouble. The Danes have a word for this ideal, '*hygge*', and when I met the Andersens and Charlotte I knew I was in a *hygge* heartland.

49

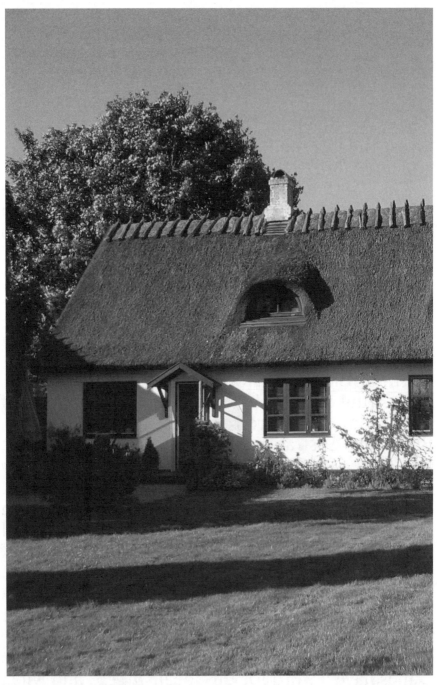

THE ANDERSEN'S FAIRYTALE HOUSE, NORTH OF
ELSINORE

Do you have an image in your mind of Hans Christian Andersen's fairytale countryside? I'm sure they're no relation but the Andersen's house fitted the bill: flowers climbing up the freshly painted white frontage, red painted nine-paned wooden windows, two symmetrical chimneys sprouting from the thatched roof which gently curved like old-fashioned beehives over two first floor windows.

Kai Andersen was building a west-facing conservatory on to the white-painted thatched cottage when I arrived. 'This will be our Florida room,' he explained in perfectly enunciated English-English. Marianne and Charlotte took me to visit the dogs who were lazing in the adjacent field.

The Broholmer is a mastiff breed, the size of a Great Dane. It became extinct early in the twentieth century and what I was seeing now was a reconstructed version, created from a variety of surviving local dogs augmented with a little help from, of all breeds, the Spanish mastiff. Macy took one look at these massive hulks, turned to me and, with her eyes said, 'I'm outta here!'

The dog breed called the Great Dane is not actually Danish. It got its English misnomer when the French naturalist Buffon called the pick of the different guarding mastiffs from northern Germany (including those from Schleswig-Holstein) 'Grand Danois'. It would have been more accurate if we had translated the name from German rather than French. To the Germans, the Great Dane is their Deutsche Dogge, Germany's national dog, but the British had a problem acknowledging that breeds we admired could

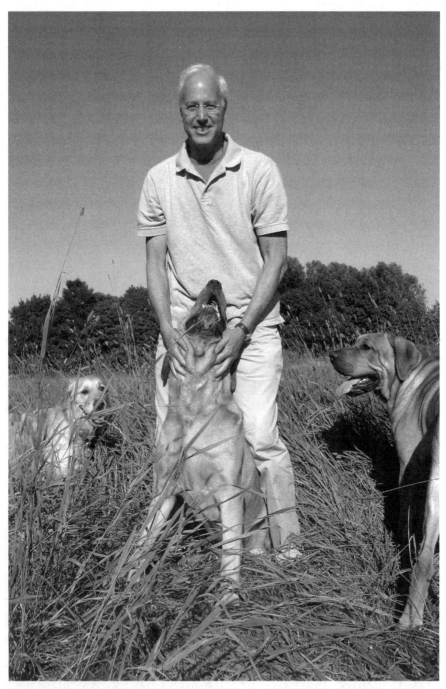

THE BROHOLMER IS A MASTIFF BREED, THE SIZE OF A GREAT DANE

actually be German. While the rest of the world called the *Deutsche Schaferhund*, the German shepherd dog, we called it the Alsatian, although the breed had no heritage in that region of (depending on the results of the most recent conflict) France or Germany.

Here in Denmark, the Broholmer served the same purpose as the Great Dane in Germany, as a guardian dog on country estates. Although the Danish Kennel Club retained a breed standard for it, the last one was registered in 1910. In the 1980s Danish breeders started a programme to recreate the breed to the original conformation standards. I was surrounded by the fruits of that programme now—tawny-coloured, black-nosed, 60 kilo hulks.

Back in the dining-room, Macy assumed her natural position under the teak table while Marianne and Charlotte and I had tea and biscuits. The Broholmers sat like bookends at either side of us. We were joined by the Andersen's daughter and boyfriend, who spoke in English to each other simply because I was there. I was invited to stay but was itchy to get going, to reach lands I'd never before visited.

We camped near Elsinore and spent much of the evening on the nearby seashore. In the woods leading to the sea I met a young couple walking their four-month-old blond Hovawart pup and as we talked the owner picked a tick off Macy's head.

'They are very common. Each time you walk in the woods she will get them,' he advised. 'There is mange from foxes too. Dogs frequently get it. Foxes have moved into central Copenhagen and even dogs there are getting the fox mange.' As we talked he noticed another small tick emerge from the hair on my dog's head. Although I had treated Macy with tick prevention before I left London, I gave her a thorough inspection before she got back in the Roadtrek, and treated her yet again. I didn't tell the Hovawart's owner he'd spotted ticks on a vet's dog, but there's a job waiting for him in London if he's interested.

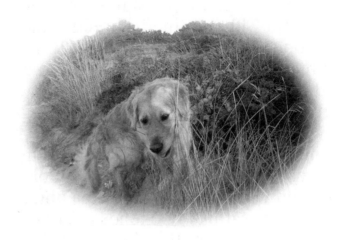

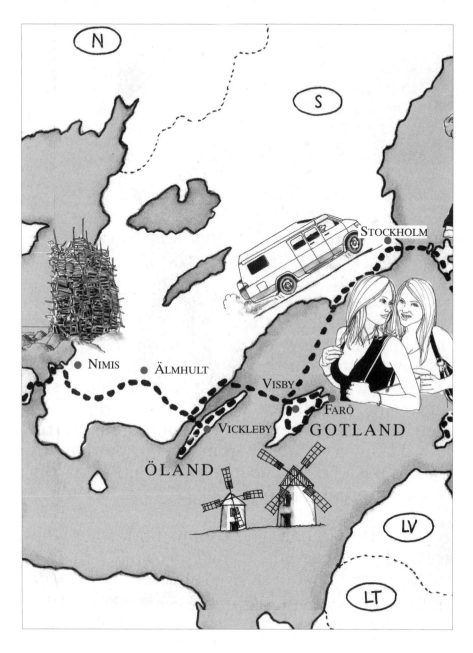

CHAPTER TWO

SWEDEN

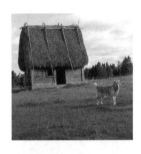

SWEDEN

People per square kilometre	*20*
Dogs per square kilometre	*1.5*
Number of Swedes killed annually by hand guns	*5*
Number of Swedes killed annually by moose	*8*

Hollyhocks were tied back to the fronts of the thatched and tiled cottages, which were red or pink or white or yellow or green or blue, but always freshly painted. In the gardens branches of apple and pear trees drooped, some almost to the grass, under the abundance of the year's crop. Fallen fruit was everywhere. Over a hundred sparrows lofted lazily into the air from a single garden as we walked past. On the nearby pink granite coastline, two cormorants sat on a jagged rock, motionless, like weathervanes.

Perfectly camouflaged comma butterflies whose colouring matched the orange-brown lichen on the rocks flitted amongst a profusion of lavender-coloured common knapweed. The old wooden sailing and fishing boats that sat motionless in the small harbour were immaculately varnished and maintained. Arild, which sits on the Kullaberg peninsula on the west coast of Sweden, was dressed to perfection, a flawless seaside village masterful in its studied carelessness.

I'd come here for a guaranteed good lunch at Rusthållargården, a local hotel and restaurant, but I had another reason for making the trip. Somewhere to the west of Arild, hidden deep in the Kullaberg Nature Reserve, was a curiously un-Swedish place—an anarchic creation, an 'independent country'. 'Nimis' is a raspberry in the face of authority, a nail that wouldn't be hammered down. At the hotel they told me how to get there, and I drove to the nature reserve, donned waterproof trousers and jacket against the rain and tramped for two hours through creeping juniper, wild honeysuckle, sloe and hawthorn, following the well-signed red-and-blue hiking routes, searching for the bloody thing.

There wasn't a single soul around to ask but just as I was about to give up, I saw a small yellow patch on a tree with a black 'N' painted on it. That sign took me off the well-tended trails deep into the trackless, sodden woods. The ground was slippery and now it became steep. Under the canopy of late summer beech and oak leaves it was so dark I couldn't see the next 'N' sign and I frequently stopped, backtracked and tried other routes. For over an hour we descended, ascended and descended more.

Macy, who usually charges through woodland with abandon, carefully took one step at a time, meticulously making the descent with conscious deliberation. Even so, at one point she loosened a rock and set a mini-avalanche cascading down the hill.

With rain dripping off my hat and glasses I thought I'd reached an impenetrable wall of woods, but suddenly there seemed to be an

57

entrance, a tunnel through the branches, tall enough to walk through, and then a staircase made of branches leading down out of the darkness to the light of the rocky coast and water below. In front of me was a driftwood tower—a matchstick lighthouse 15 metres high—and another tower, and another.

They stretched away into the distance, and it was so disorientating that I couldn't judge the size of the furthest ones, but then, high in one tower I saw movement and heard a man speaking German on his mobile phone. Driftwood walkways five metres above ground connected one tower to another. When the tide was high, the distant towers at the water's edge must be surrounded by surf.

The sight was stunning, mad and arrestingly beautiful; when I saw it I knew absolutely that art needn't be restricted to galleries and museums. These chaotic, towering driftwood structures don't clash with nature, this is art as a creative component of nature. I was mesmerised. As the rain fell steadily, I sat there wondering what went through the maker's mind—what primordial impulse compelled him to build here? Was it a desire to show that nature and culture are wholly compatible?

It was obvious that Nimis had become, at least in part, art as entertainment, with visitors roaming the towers and walkways like an adventure playground, but had the artist considered that?

There's more to Nimis, and the place has a curious history and has come to symbolise something more than its aesthetic value. It's become a *cause célèbre*, encouraged, magnified,

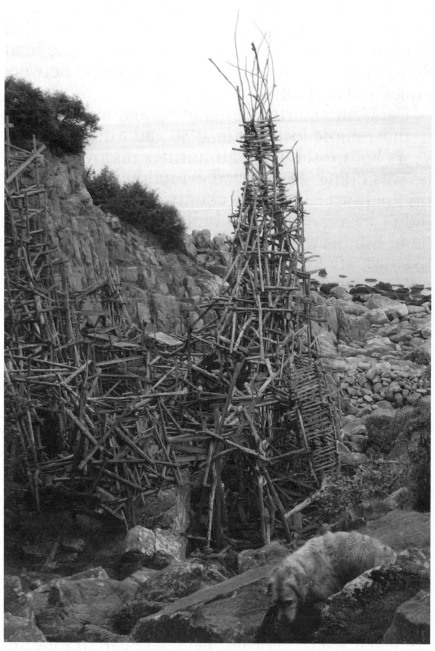

A TOWER IN THE 'INDEPENDENT COUNTRY' OF
NIMIS

and even defined through interaction with the media. Did its creator think that art could become a form of guerrilla warfare with authority? Did he know, when he embarked on this venture that, here in supremely conformist 'don't rock the boat' Sweden, he was setting a collision course between ethics and aesthetics?

Lars Vilks started hammering and nailing Nimis in this remote location in 1980 and worked for two years before the local authorities discovered what he was doing. He carried everything to the site in his knapsack. The local county council told him he didn't have a licence to build and ordered him to demolish his work and when he didn't, it took him to court. He lost.

He appealed to the district court, and lost. He appealed to Sweden's supreme court, and lost, each time being fined more and more kronor. Vilks then hatched a cunning plan. If he was simply the artist, not the owner, he couldn't be compelled to tear down his creation. He sold Nimis to the German artist Joseph Beuys and when Beuys died it became the property of the conceptual artist Christo. The Swedish authorities now found themselves in argument with one of the most successful and respected conceptual artists of the twentieth century.

By then Nimis had grown into a massive work of art—over twenty-five tons of wood, tens of towers over a hundred metres of coastline. What I was looking at now, notwithstanding intermittent vandalism by fire and chain saw, or the work of ferocious winter storms, weighed over 70 tons and stretches over 150 metres along the shore.

In 1991, Vilks started another project, 'Arx',

building more towers using concrete and stones. Again, he carried everything to the site in his knapsack but this time round, challenges from the authorities had become part of his art. Describing Arx as a 352-page 'book in stone', he arranged through a publishing house to sell 'pages'. Arx suddenly had over 300 owners. The county council backed off, deciding that the matter should be dealt with by the landowner, who decided to do nothing. To err on the side of safety, and to add additional protection to his 'art', Vilks created the independent country of Ladonia and proclaimed Nimis and Arx to be protected national monuments.

Traditional art—painting and sculpture—is simple. It's moveable and has a value. Art is objects. Art endures. Vilks plays with that concept of art—something that's entertaining to me but doubtless highly irritating to others—and Nimis is as much a philosophy as it is a grand artistic creation. Art has value but Nimis, by the very nature of its location and what it stands for, has no material worth at all. Vilks' chosen museum is the Kullaberg Nature Reserve, not an endowed institution in an urban conurbation. The maintenance work is constant. When Vilks ceases to hammer and nail—and he's gone through 160,000 nails so far—his 'art' will disintegrate and disappear. The local county council he fought with for 25 years, Höganäs Kommun, now highlights Nimis on its website as a must-see tourist highlight and boasts that 30,000 people visited last year. They must all visit in July and August because, apart from the German guy, I was the only other human in the Kullaberg Nature Reserve that day.

Macy and I climbed back up the cliffs and through the woods. My heart was beating in my ears, 160 beats a minute. Even Macy was stopping, collecting her thoughts and strength, then proceeding. Later, when I checked a rock-climbing website to see the degree of difficulty of that walk, it was classified as a '3', which means 'entering the realm of scrambling, going up an incline over a rough/rocky terrain, not quite necessitating the use of hands to maintain balance and forward progression.' Rubbish. I joined Macy using all fours to clamber back up the rocky and greasy slope.

I can't recommend the nature reserve as a great place to camp overnight because if I did I'd be contravening Höganäs Kommun rules. Obeying rules is, after all, part of Swedish DNA. Sweden does have an excellent unwritten convention called 'Allemans ratt'—the right of common access—that permits anyone to walk anywhere, to camp or spend the night anywhere, as long as you don't infringe upon the privacy of home owners or damage the property you stay on, but there's one exception, and that's nature reserves. At dusk the rain abated. Macy snapped at mosquitoes while I made a tomato omelette, then a delicious pear sauce from windfall fruit I'd collected in Arild, and warm cheese crackers.

CRISPY CHEESE CRACKERS
Using a Swedish cheese slicer, slice thin sheets of cheese off a block of hard Västerbotten cheese. Heat a frying pan until warm-hot then place the cheese slices side by side in the pan, covering the bottom.

As they melt, the slices will meld together. As soon as small bubbles of air burst holes in the cheese, remove the frying pan from the heat and gently tilt it on to absorbent paper kitchen roll.
Allow the thin wafer of savoury, salty cheese to cool and go crispy.
Break into bits and eat with warm, sweet, pear sauce.

I enjoy visiting Sweden because it's so easy to turn my brain off here, relax and take in the scenery. While its neighbours, Norway, Denmark and Finland, all suffered from the twentieth century's wars, Sweden hasn't experienced border changes or blood loss for generations. I headed for Älmhult, buried in the dense forests in Småland, where friends live.

Älmhult is home to the first-ever IKEA and so Swedes say that's where Father Christmas really comes from. The sun had reappeared, but I couldn't take much advantage of the good weather and explore the countryside. The risk-averse Swedes long ago installed hideous moose fencing along all main Swedish highways, and though that means they've successfully reduced road deaths from moose accidents it sure makes it difficult to stop for a walk in the woods.

Occasionally I'd pull on to a side-road and we'd stroll through conifer woodland carpeted in deer moss. I picked blueberries, which were scarce; either these areas had been trawled by Baltic and Polish pickers employed by Swedes to do this menial work, or it simply hadn't been a good year for blueberries.

I was now in the Earth's northernmost forest,

the boreal forest, a continuous belt of woodland that encircles the globe. I felt utterly at home. Seventy-three per cent of it is in the Russian Federation but 22 per cent lies in Canada, where I camped and canoed as a boy. The Nordic countries contain the remaining five per cent. Eight months previously, when I was last here, a local hurricane-force winter storm decimated a small dot of the boreal forest: 300,000,000 trees snapped like matchsticks or were torn from the ground. This book could very well be printed on paper from those storm-uprooted trees in Småland.

The Gustafssons, with whom I'd be staying the night, lost half the trees across the road from their home. The forest where Lars Gustafsson's parents lived was turned into an impenetrable maze of fallen trees, inaccessible for days, even to walkers. To the rest of the world the Småland storm was a non-event but to the Gustafssons it was a cold breath of death.

The woods along the roads to Älmhult looked as if they had been untidily logged out; everywhere there were enormous piles of cut timber. Everywhere I drove there were snakes of thick black hose pumping water over the serried ranks of logs. Outside Ljungby at a mothballed airport there was a 2200-metre long, 75-metre wide pile of 4,000,000 trees. Later I learned it was the largest log pile in the world. Over 80,000 people had arrived in the last few months just to gawk at it. The amount of water needed to prevent that log pile from spontaneous combustion was enough to service a town of 50,000 people.

Dried, blackened lupin stalks lined the verges of

the road. In springtime the Swedish countryside is overwhelmed by their purple stocks. They are indigenous to the Mediterranean, but the Swedes planted them on degraded forest soils to enhance nitrogen recycling, and they then 'escaped' and now thrive wherever soil has been freshly turned—especially along new highways and rail lines. At IKEA I bought sheets to fit my now enormous bed, an extra pillow, a folding wooden chair and a pasta strainer and drove on to spend the rest of the day with the Gustafssons.

There's a rough Swedish equivalent to the Danish *'hygge'*—*'trevlig'*—and that permeates life here. It's a hard word to translate into English but the longer you spend in this land, the more you understand it as an approach to life. Something that is *'trevlig'* is familiar, wholesome, cosy, accommodating, reassuring, simple, uncomplicated, unexaggerated, basic, functional, practical, attractive, intimate. Candlelight is *trevlig*. *Pepparkaka and glögg*—gingerbread and mulled wine—are *trevlig*. So is gathering around a log fire, going for a sleigh ride, having a picnic in the garden, eating food you have grown or raised or collected yourself.

Once, while eating at the Madonna Restaurant in Venice, a nearby table of young men in jackets and ties broke into song. They were a Swedish male voice choir. They produced quite simply the most beautiful music ever, not only because of where we were, but also because *'trevlig'* infuses their soft, lilting, tonal language. It's in Swedish interior design, their cooking, their gardening, even in the *Systema naturae*, the rational, logical, sensible, international language created 200 years

65

ago by a Swede from Småland, Carl Von Linne, now the *lingua franca* of twitchers, gardeners, zoologists and botanists.

The German *'gemütlichkeit'* or Dutch *'gezelligheid'* come close to matching it, but are not so all-inclusive. Christmas is the high season of *trevlig*. It's the most enchanting time of year in Sweden, especially if you're a visitor and know you don't have to stay for the rest of the winter.

Lars and Kristina Gustafsson are a twenty-first century Swedish couple with two young boys and they live in *trevliga* isolation half an hour north of Älmhult. Lars' parents had an even simpler, more isolated lifestyle, of the type rapidly passing into history. They spoke no English, lived deep in the woods in great seclusion and relied wholly upon their own physical strength and abilities to earn a living. Their son, Lars, and his wife, Kristina, may appear to live a bumpkin kind of life but bumpkins they are not. When Julia and I last stayed with them earlier this year in their forever being restored Victorian gingerbread house, I came upstairs for dinner, Lars took one look at me in a cashmere jumper and brown cords and said, 'You look just like a Long Island orthodontist.' Kristina had just completed her doctoral thesis on the barriers to integration of Muslim women into Swedish culture.

This time we talked about antiques while the kids grabbed hunks of Macy's hair, and about where I was travelling, and about the rotation of Angolans, Bosnians and Iraqis who now visit Lars' ailing father to cook and clean for him. We talked about the great Småland storm and, over delicious beets baked like potatoes on a bed of sea salt, we talked quietly and privately about Lars' mother who had frozen to death in that storm, when she ventured out to seek help for her husband.

*   *   *

Sweden was the largest country I visited on the journey and I lazed my way through it. Småland is virtually all lakes and forest now, but 150 years ago it was more intensely farmed and densely populated. Famine drove people to leave in their tens of thousands, mostly for Minnesota and Wisconsin. Their great-grandchildren return as tourists in such prodigious numbers that genealogical research has become one of the region's most successful tourist attractions.

Each day I'd wake early and squash as many of the mosquitoes that had somehow evaded the screened windows and entered the inner sanctum of the Roadtrek as I could, then breakfast and spend the day meandering to my next stop. It was cooler now but the air was crystal clear and the waters still warm enough for invigorating swimming. At one deep blue lake where I stopped for coffee and a soak in the sunshine, Macy joyously splashed in the sandy shallows, charging at ducks that nonchalantly skated away from her into the adjacent reeds. Just offshore a large lean fish, probably a pike, leapt into the air, snapped its jaws and crashed back into the crisp water. Sitting by the blue-black sweet waters of those lakes was like a homecoming. It wasn't just a visual echo of the lakes where I grew up in Ontario, it was a scent and sound reminder too. There's a comforting solitude in being alone in such beauty. But I

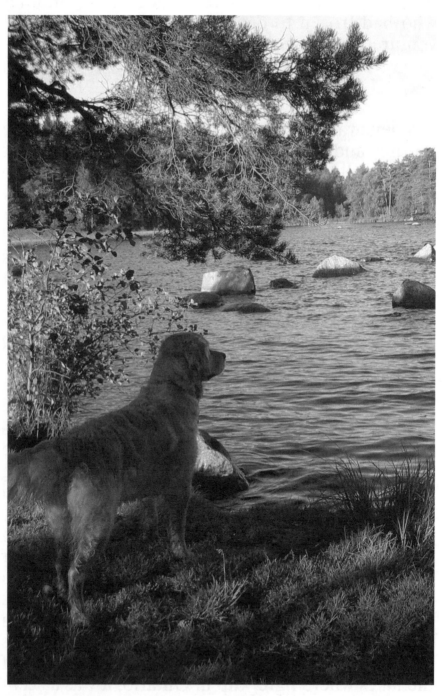

One of the many lakes in Småland

wished Julia was with me.

*   *   *

There were three squashed hedgehogs on the
road heading north on Öland; although I was only
six kilometres away from the east coast of Sweden
I was in a strikingly different terrain with its
own local ecology, a Baltic-influenced natural
history. Hedgehogs are virtually unheard of in
neighbouring mainland Småland. After driving
past piles of recently harvested sugar beets and
potatoes, I wandered through ancient coastal hay
meadows, through eyebright, milkwort and grasses
I'd never seen before, down towards the west-
facing beach. There were no mosquitoes.

While an eagle floated in the sky above, I sat in
the meadow grass and thought that in a curious
way this island was reminiscent of the Orkneys.
Both have ancient human histories as old as or
older than the mainland itself, that reveal
themselves in the way farms are still laid out, and
in the way this fragile land has been altered
through thousands of years of intensive use.

Öland itself is nowhere more than 16 kilometres
wide but at 137 kilometres long it's the fourth
largest island in the Baltic Sea. I'd been to the
north of Öland before, through its pastures,
woods, and coastal landscape of limestone pillars
weathered by the sea into natural sculptures. Near
Borgholm I stopped at a hotel restaurant for a
light lunch, wild mushroom soup, peppered goats'
cheese, local strawberry sorbet and coffee.

French cooking might concentrate on technique
but Swedish cooking is about aesthetics, texture

and *trevlig*. It's minimalist, almost Japanese in the importance of its neat, sometimes austere, presentation. It's about local produce, seafood, freshwater food, forest food and game, and I love it.

That evening I camped near chocolate-box Vickleby where the Swedish designer Carl Malmsten set up Capellagården, a commune-like craft and design school. Malmsten said that both art and the creation of art should stimulate the mind, body and soul. Julia, who deals in Swedish antiques, once had a striking pair of simple, 1930s' gloss black, wooden candlesticks that looked like urns. They were designed by Malmsten, and spoke just as he had intended his creations to do. I regret that she sold them.

Of course, there were small, rickety windmills everywhere, often in rows of three or more. They have become Öland's USP, on every tourist brochure. There's also the Great Alvar Plain, a pavement-like limestone barren that covers most of the south of the island, devoid of trees but covered by black, orange and green lichens, mosses and grasses, is the largest of its kind in the world—15 kilometres wide and well over 37 kilometres long. Alvars are plant communities on limestone flats whose shallow soil is very alkaline and favours mosses and herbs. The Scandinavian alvars are the world's best known, although I spent my childhood summers on what geologists (but few others) call the 'Carden Alvar', a region of thin limestone soil and alkaline lakes east of Lake Simcoe in Ontario.

It was now mid-September and I saw blue butterflies—Large Blues, I think—over the alvar.

It was a surprise to see such a fragile species of insect—they've been extinct in Britain for years—in such a northerly location and so late in the year.

There were plump flycatchers too, stopover birds resting and refuelling before flying on to Italy, another stopover on their way back to Africa after summering in the Arctic. This desolate, haunting region had once been intensively farmed too. Drystone walls, built to keep livestock and wild animals away from cultivated crops, divided the land but now the thin soil nourished nothing higher than blue fruiting juniper bushes. Here and there were granite boulders, deposited on the plain during the last Ice Age.

Local literature told me that in the wooded northern part of the Ottenby Nature Reserve near the southern end of Öland there are 200 fallow deer, descendants of deer transported here over 300 years ago when the whole island was the Swedish king's private hunting ground. Generally speaking I trust what the law-abiding Swedes say (although I have to say that I learned early on that some Swedish antique dealers are positively Italianate in their ability to create genuine 'antiques') so I believe the literature when it says that until 1801 it was illegal for a peasant to keep a dog lest it chase the king's wildlife. I started to feel a little sceptical, however, when I read that peasants could keep dogs if they amputated one of the dog's front legs. How did they do that? Do you know how big those front leg arteries are?

Occasionally, after a road traffic accident, or because of the growth of a cancer that can only be cured through radical surgery, I'm forced to amputate a dog's leg. The surgery is fairly mechanical. Dogs don't have scapulas so there's no bone attachment to the body, only muscles. The surgery is really dissection combined with blood vessel ligating. Maybe there were lots of canine amputees populating this Swedish province 200 years ago but it's virtually guaranteed that, for cultural reasons, you won't come across a three-legged dog today, either here or anywhere else in Sweden.

In the UK, 33 per cent of the dog population is over ten years old. In Germany over 35 per cent of dogs are ten or over. In Sweden only 17 per cent of dogs fall within this age band. It's not because veterinary care in Sweden in poor—Swedish veterinary medicine is equal to the best anywhere. There aren't many old dogs, and there are no three-legged dogs as a result of the powerful conformist streak in the Swedish national culture.

Let me explain. The first time I saw a Gustavian country house or 'herrgård' I was enchanted by the symmetry of the building, and I wanted to live in it. It wasn't long before I discovered that I could have one just like it—there were identical country houses everywhere. Virtually every single country house built in the late 1700s and early 1800s, the 'Gustavian' period, was similar: rectangular, three storeys high, a central doorway at the front and a matching door at the back leading to the garden, two large windows and tall, tiled, wood burning 'kakelugns' in each room.

Regardless of your status in society in the Gustavian period, you conformed to what was expected of you. Your house must be similar to that of your equals, even if you were the local landowner. No more. No less. The impact on the

Swedish psyche was deep. That compulsion to conform is still pervasive.

Drive through the Swedish countryside and its apparent that not only are most pre-twentieth century homes painted the same '*Falu* red', but they are also designed and constructed similarly. Conformist culture also affects the decisions that dog owners make. They turn down the offer of radiation therapy or chemotherapy or amputations for their pets, not because they love their dogs any less than we do but because they can't help but consider, 'What would the neighbours think?'

I'm not saying that radical treatments should always be undertaken to treat life-threatening health problems in pets. There are some canine personalities that cope badly with intensive treatments and it can be selfish on our part to make a dog endure them when we're really doing it for ourselves, not our pets. But the decision on whether or not to engage in that radical treatment should be made by asking whether a dog will suffer from either the treatment or the consequences of the treatment. If it won't, then why not give it the opportunity of a longer life?

Vets who perform amputations know that amputees can thrive and that radiation or chemotherapy can be benign experiences for pets because regimes are created to ensure a low likelihood of adverse reactions. Macy's life expectancy is greater, not because of her genes, not because of the quality of veterinary care available for her, but because she lives permanently in Britain, not Sweden.

*   *   *

73

'Your vehicle gives me goose bumps,' he explained when I saw him gazing at my Roadtrek. 'It reminds me of British Columbia.'

Hilmar-Lutz and his wife Elizabeth came from Sieseby in northern Germany and were on their way, with their bicycles and their lanky black-and-tan dog Fiona, from Oskarshamn on Sweden's east coast, to Gotland, the Baltic Sea's most isolated large island. Of all the ferry journeys so far this was by far the most civilised. Not only do the Destination Gotland ferries cruise at close to 30 knots, making the 90 kilometre journey through the Baltic Sea in well under three hours, they also provide a *trevliga* lounge exclusively for dogs and their owners.

It was only after Macy and I had taken our seats in the dog lounge that I learned the local protocol. You bring your dog's blanket, bed and water bowl up from your car for the journey. Elizabeth immediately offered her dog's full water bowl to Macy who emptied it in seconds. 'He never gives me a drink,' she explained with mournful eyes.

The Posers were in love with Canada, but more recently they'd been spending time closer to home, in Europe's nearest equivalent. They visited Sweden often. When I commented on their superb English—in my presence, like the Andersens, they spoke English to each other—Hilmar-Lutz explained that English has other uses. When they travelled a few kilometres from their home to visit Denmark, they only spoke English. 'They still remember 1868,' he twinkled, mentioning the year when the Prussians officially made Schleswig-Holstein their own. Hilmar-Lutz twinkled a lot. He has a gentle face, a perfect attribute for a family general practitioner, although he was in fact a radiologist.

So we talked medicine. I learned that Fiona, lying on her blanket at their feet was on medication for a dilated heart condition and I commented on my experience with the drug she was being given. That sure perked up the other dog owners around us, all Swedes. In perfect English they told me the medical histories of their dogs.

The champagne-coloured golden retriever to my right, a bitch that frequently tried to climb on to her owner's lap, had only one oestrus cycle a year and dodgy hips. The owner of the two miniature schnauzers to my left had a third dog that died at three years of age from a tick-transmitted disease. Elsewhere in the '*djursalong*' (the 'animal lounge') were two more golden retrievers, a poodle, a Samoyed, two middle schnauzers, two dachshunds, a Labrador, a border terrier, two Irish wolfhounds, a boxer and a Vasgotaspets. Not a crossbreed mutt in sight. Not a surprise in responsible Sweden where unauthorised canine assignations are as rare as three-legged dogs.

Hilmar-Lutz and I talked a little politics. (Swedes don't find that kind of thing *trevlig*.) The Posers were worried about Germany's future.

'We received our voting papers and still do not know who to vote for. I feel none of the parties, the Reds, the Blacks, even the Greens, have a realistic vision of the future. We must be pragmatic and plan ahead. That means a drop in our living standards.' I also learned that his grandfather,

75

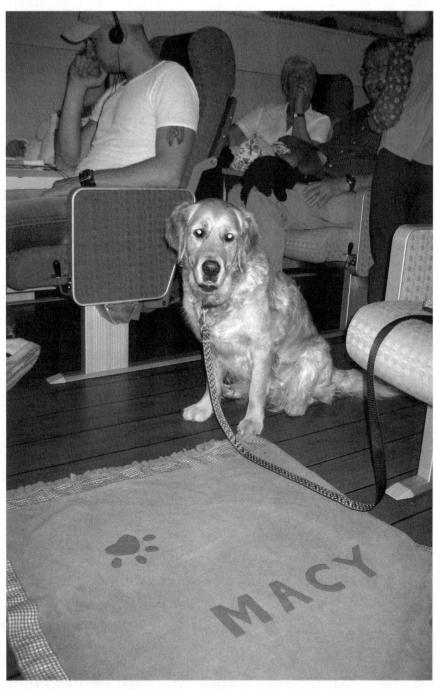

Lounge protocol on the Gotland ferry

Max Frey, had been a veterinarian to the famous Lutz Heck, the curator of the Berlin Zoo. Heck was a self-proclaimed reviver of extinct breeds and the author of *Animals—My Adventure*. I've had an English translation of it for years.

*   *   *

The ferry docked on Gotland at the medieval, walled town of Visby, and I headed to the northern tip of the island and across the narrow Farosund strait by ferry to Farö or Sheep Island, passing a British military cemetery near Ryssnas, on my way to Sudersand for an afternoon swim in the late summer sunshine. The cemetery was the final resting place for British sailors, victims of cholera in the 1850s, when the British navy was based in Farosund before it advanced with the French navy upon Russia during the Crimean War.

On the sandy beach there were cockle, clam and two types of mussel shells, black sea mussels and white Baltic ones, all surprisingly small. Clinging to the rocks beneath where I swam were thousands and thousands of miniature black sea mussels, nothing else, and none more than three centimetres long. The water tasted like August freshwater, like lake water that had been heated through the summer.

The Baltic's waters themselves are replenished by rivers and fresh-water runoff from the surrounding lands—very little seawater funnels into it through the narrow Øresund between Denmark and Sweden and the Danish Store Bælt. The result is low salinity, 0.5 per cent compared to the North Sea's 3.5 per cent. Few true sea

77

creatures can survive and, if they do, as the sea mussel does, their growth is often stunted. They proliferate though, as there are no sea stars or shore crabs to threaten their numbers, as there are on the Øresund side of the Sweden peninsula. Here, only flounder and eider ducks devour them.

Across the sound, Farö had a tough, harsh beauty. I hadn't expected anywhere in Sweden to look like this. The landscape around Langhammarshammar on the west side of Farö is almost Iberian in its barrenness, but for an occasional, isolated, stunted, wind-racked pine that survives the westerly winter gales off the Baltic. Dry limestone walls separated the fields and small limestone windmills, some converted to summer cottages, dotted the fields between the compact farm buildings.

Grey, hornless Gotland sheep, raised for their wool, grazed all but the thistles from their pastures. Juniper bushes by the edge of the fields were stripped as high as the sheep could reach. This is the driest and the sunniest region anywhere in Sweden. I slept that night to the gentle sound of waves rolling on to the shingle beach and awoke once more to a cloudless, crisp but warm day.

The morning sea was as smooth as glass, the sloping shingle beach of reef limestone blindingly white and the tall, slender sea stacks in the water and on the shore were like trolls' tombstones and, I bet, an inspiration for Lars Vilks' Nimis. Black-backed gulls cruised the shoreline while Macy fought for her footing on the shingle then took to the water.

The entire island is composed of fossilised shells and skeletons of marine organisms over

400 million years old. You don't have to crack rocks open to get at them. I saw fossilised button corals lying at the base of a sea stack. Further up the beach, the shingle looked darker, then almost black with covering lichen. From a distance the coastal landscape looked sterile, but for those gnarled Scots pine, but there amongst the white shingle grew tall, yellow flowering, long-leafed, woad plants, once the source of the Vikings' blue dye.

I came across a profusion of little wild geraniums, purple-flowered Herb Robert. At the top of the beach, just beyond the road was a windswept pine forest and beneath it a carpet of Alpine bearberry. Some of the bearberry leaves were turning to their autumn colour and would soon turn the forest floor a defiant crimson. There were isolated clumps of seaweed on the shore. Yesterday, approaching the Nature Reserve, I saw seaweed being loaded on to a tractor trailer. The old tradition of using seaweed to fertilise the soil must still be practised here, if only by Swedes holidaying at their Gotland summer homes.

At Digerhuvud I made breakfast looking out over hundreds of sea stacks and while I was there, a Volvo arrived and the woman passenger unfolded a chair, sat down and started knitting with grey wool. Her husband, an immaculately kitted-out fisherman in green waders, green fishing jacket and green hat, made his way to the beach. She told me this was a perfect spot for *'torsk'* fishing—cod fishing—and she was certain that was what they would be eating for dinner. While we talked, Macy disappeared amongst the sea stacks on the rocky beach and returned triumphant with a plastic bottle in her mouth, doing her bit to keep Farö's beaches tidy.

On the back roads we passed perfectly restored stone walls, pristine farm buildings and farmhouses with well-tended gardens. Lars had described Farö as a remote suburb of affluent Stockholmers and now I understood what he meant. There was serious money—urban money— spent in these austere barrens.

I drove past a flower-filled meadow with pollarded trees and we stopped for a walk in a natural bonanza: the meadow was a carpet of azure-blue cornflowers amongst which stood ancient pollarded crab apple and hawthorn trees, all less than three metres high. This glade was once harvested not only for herbs and grasses but also for branches and leaves to use as winter fodder for livestock. Hay-making and pollarding in one location—unusual, though it makes excellent sense.

The meadow was replenished every year by the moult of fallen leaves. In spring, when the wood anemone—locals still call it the 'raking flower'— was in bloom, the meadow was raked of the last of the fallen twigs and remaining leaves. Fresh hay sprouted. The field I was in must have been cut at least a month before, tended and turned weekly, just as I had seen near Arnhem in the Netherlands. The second harvest of pollarded spindly twigs and thin branches had yet to be made and judging from the profuse growth of thin, upright branches it would be a plentiful one.

Near the free ferry back to Gotland Macy and I visited a sedge-thatched sheep shelter—the wonderful local word for the shelter is *'lammgift'*—

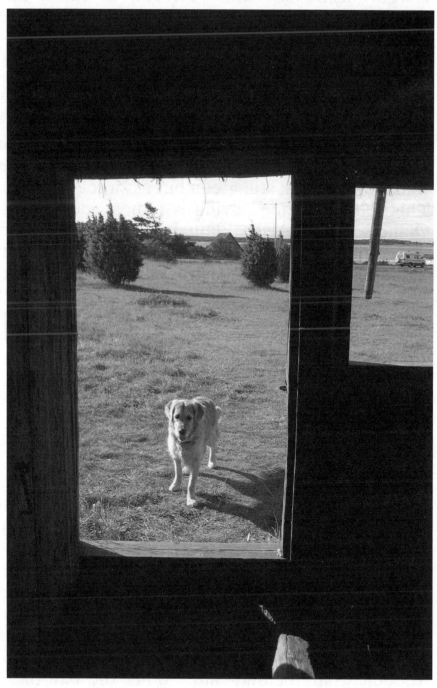

MACY TURNED DOWN THE INVITATION TO ENTER THE '*LAMMGIFT*'

I went inside but Macy refused to enter, and entertained herself by chewing on a discarded plank.

*   *   *

Back in north-west Gotland the landscape was slighter lusher but still a spartan combination of juniper bushes and Scots pine scrubland. I picked wild strawberries, still green but as sweet as honey. This flat limestone paving is almost identical to Øland's Great Alvar Plain but far, far smaller. Green moss and orange lichen grew in patches on the limestone while from cracks in the pavement, scraggly pines strove to survive. There was a carpet of succulent leafed, yellow flowering stonecrop and everywhere a host of centimetre-long, red-and-black firebugs resting on the leathery leaves of Vincetoxicum. They reminded me of my childhood in Ontario where firebugs, on hot summer days, feed on toxic milkweed plants.

*   *   *

A side-road took us along the east coast of Gotland, by a bay as smooth as a millpond. Standing tall and erect at a stainless steel table, gutting flounder by the water's edge was a man of the sea. In the mid-morning sunshine his red rubber apron glistened. His unpainted wooden fishing boat, with a small motor, oars, nets, floats and pennants on a long pole was docked at a wooden wharf behind him. Along the bay there were fields of strikingly shaped sea-stacks mushrooming amongst the shrubs and trees and ground-covering rock roses. I stopped at the man's smokery for some smoked *'flundra'* and *'lax'*, turbot and salmon. He also sold *'torsk file'* or cod fillets, *'gadda'* and *'sik'*—pike and whitefish—both freshwater creatures that survive, even thrive, in the low salinity of the Baltic.

The smoker didn't speak English, or German, or even Swedish unless prodded. He quietly went about his business and I got the feeling that it was more of an inconvenience than a sales opportunity to deal with me and the driver of another car that stopped.

'Vad kostar?' I asked

'Hundra fem,' he replied. I got no more words out of him.

Behind the row of rustic, unpainted fishermen's cabins, boat-houses and docks lining the edge of the bay was an old grey 1980s' Buick Monte Carlo—the smoker's car, similar to the last vehicle my father owned. I wanted to take a photo of him, standing upright at his work table, preparing his catch for the smoker but was embarrassed to ask such a dignified individual. Driving away, it occurred to me that I saw my father in this man and he would have just loved having his photo taken.

Where fields or shores on Gotland beckoned I pulled over and let Macy shoot off after rabbits or hares. Rabbits, introduced in the twentieth century, flourished, were decimated by myxomatosis, flourished again and in the last 10 years have been decimated once more, this time by rabbit haemorrhagic disease. No one knows exactly how these virus infections made their way to this isolated island but it's commonly believed they were intentionally introduced by farmers hoping to control the destructive rabbit population. Mace was here to help.

Blue-flowered chicory was studded with tall marguerites and late poppies added their colour. Macy rolled in a field that was like a plantation of cornflowers, blossoming after the wheat had been harvested, as if in a defiant last stand against our intervention. Holstein-Friesians, ubiquitous everywhere in northern Europe, grazed between milkings on the pastureland.

I visited several of Gotland's 92 churches and was reminded that even 800 years ago, long before the Gustavian era, conformity ran deep in the hearts of these people. All the churches were built between 1000, when Christianity came to the island and 1350, when the Gotland economy collapsed, leaving the churches frozen in time, and it was hard to distinguish between them.

All of these limestone churches were of a classic three-part division, each with its window behind the altar, facing east. Some of the churches were Romanesque, with intricately carved portals, round arches and barrel vaults but most had been rebuilt in Gothic style, with pointed arches and ribbed vaults. With their sharply pointed spires, even the tiniest of them has an almost ethereal verticality as if the church itself were aspiring towards heaven.

As I returned to the Roadtrek after visiting Bal church, which for some inexplicable reason was surrounded by myriad firebugs, I saw a tick walking across Macy's forehead. I gave her a thorough search and applied more deterrent. At Bro church, I was entranced by the rustic, painted baptismal font and wall paintings and Macy was bewitched by the odours from the pews. We walked in the pine woods nearby and it dawned on me that elsewhere in Sweden the floor of pine forests consists of lichens, ferns, lingonberries, blueberries and low brush but here on Gotland the ground was thick with grasses and cow parsley. On the road back to Visby as I passed a farm with its midsummer arch still up at its entrance, crows picked at a road-kill hedgehog.

When Visby was the commercial centre of the Hanseatic League it was one of the wealthiest cities in all of Europe, and that's why there is such a treasury of Gothic churches in so small a region. When the Baltic herring shoals mysteriously relocated themselves to the North Sea in the fourteenth century, the Hanseatic League started an inexorable decline, and was replaced by the Netherlands as the entrepôt centre of northern Europe.

Visby itself was devoid of tourists when I passed back through it. The season was over. Macy and I walked the empty, narrow, cobbled streets, and I bought some local honey and fresh baked bread, then stopped for coffee and cake. Macy was immediately given a bowl of water, and while she gravitated to four women at the adjacent table I met a local man, retired from Bromma, outside Stockholm, walking his three-month-old springer spaniel so that his wife could manage a little serious late-summer gardening.

Because we were both 'dog people' he told me that at nearby Ladbyskibet is the grave of a tenth-century Viking chieftain and that his dog is buried with him. I asked him why he had chosen to retire to the middle of the Baltic and he explained that for him it was like stepping back into his childhood. 'The churches here are not locked,' he said and the intense look in his eyes told me that that fact encapsulated everything good about Gotland.

I took the ferry back to the mainland, arriving at Nynäshamn near Stockholm, a hundred miles north up the coast from Oskarshamn, where we had left for Gotland but this time Macy travelled in the *djursalong* with her own bedding and bowls.

*   *   *

In a Stockholm park an impossibly beautiful 25-year-old girl, square, bronzed shoulders, thin, white, halter top over red bra straps, marine-blue eyes, flaxen blonde hair, smiled at me and I had to put on my sunglasses to protect myself from the blinding glare from her impossibly white, tombstone-straight teeth. Macy issued me an obedience command to stop staring. I lifted my jaw from the ground and tried to act cool. She was quite simply the most stunning woman I think I'd ever met, or was it because I'd now been living with a dog for several weeks?

She smiled at me for the same reason the Visby springer spaniel owner had talked to me, because like me she was a 'dog person' and she was exercising fat 'Rastus', her own golden retriever. Rastus took one sniff of Macy, determined that she wasn't intending to ovulate today and wandered off. Although his owner called him back he was more interested in the scent on a nearby bush. I got down on my knees and begged him to

86

come back but he didn't so she put her iPod back in her ears and jogged on.

Macy and I had lunch with Jenny and Anna, Swedish friends of my youngest daughter Tamara, in warm sunshine on an outdoor terrace in the park, overlooking the water. The girls had moved back to Sweden for work and family reasons. Jenny works in human resources for a multinational. 'It's surprising,' she explained, 'how different each culture is around the Baltic. The Finns, they are easy to do business with. All you have to do is occasionally ask, "Are you awake?" and they say yes and agree with whatever is being discussed. The Danes are much more pompous. They can be arrogant and argumentative. It's like they have a chip on their shoulder or something.'

That evening I stayed with friends in Vaxholm, north of Stockholm. Ulla prepared dinner: grilled *strömming* (Baltic herring that are smaller than North Sea herring), new potatoes, yellow beans and tomatoes, all the vegetables from her garden, and a scrumptious plum flan, the aroma of which suffused the kitchen. Åke, her husband, who teaches at the Swedish veterinary faculty at Uppsala, joined us later.

I told them I was going to travel through the Baltic states and Åke explained that after World War Two almost half of all the artificial insemination vets in Sweden were Estonian vets escaping the Russian take-over.

'You must be very careful,' Ulla interjected. 'This summer there were many camper robberies here in Sweden. It can be very dangerous to camp alone. The police say that some of the robberies are carried out by Lithuanian gangs.'

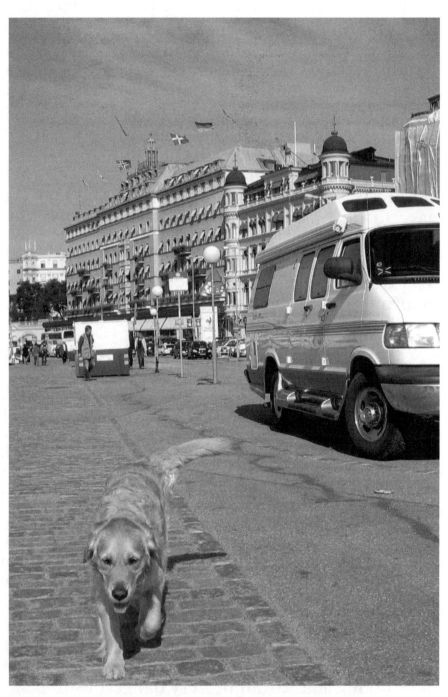

Macy goes exploring in Stockholm

Åke and Ulla have a Border terrier, Mira, who shared her floor with Macy for two days but I was more interested in another breed—a recent immigrant to Sweden, still unknown in Britain, a 'Communist dog'. I wanted to meet a Black terrier, developed, it is said, to prove that Communism could be inherited. Åke arranged for me to visit a local kennel.

*   *   *

Trofion Denisovich Lysenko was one of the twentieth century's greatest charlatans. He may, also, have been responsible for as many Russians deaths as all those who died in Russia's war with Germany. Lysenko was still alive when I started in veterinary practice, when I married, and even when my youngest child was born.

Lysenko's great deceit was to deny the truth of Mendelian genetics, and to convince the Communist Party leaders that he, Lysenko, knew the real truth about genetic inheritance and that western scientists were wrong. During his lifetime genetic research was virtually banned in the Soviet Union. Only science that was acceptable to government ideology was permitted.

What is the principle behind Mendelian genetics? Any student of basic biology knows the story of Father Gregor Mendel's common garden peas. In the 1860s, at the Augustinian abbey in Brno, Moravia (now in the Czech Republic), Mendel had been cross-pollinating green peas, concentrating on reproducing specific characteristics such as height and colour. He established that some characteristics such as

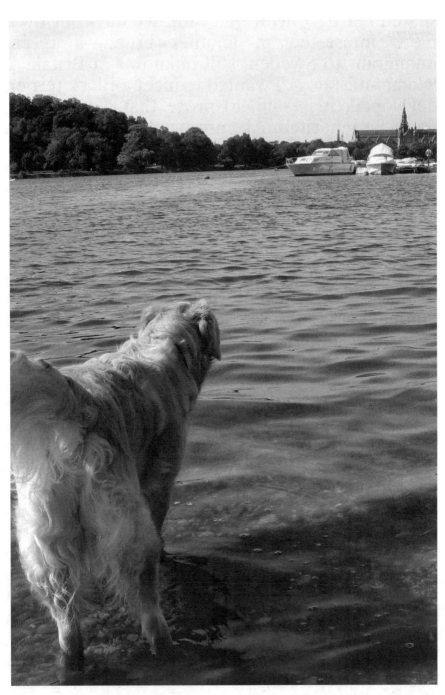

MACY IN STOCKHOLM

colour were either 'dominant' or 'recessive' and that it was possible to predict inheritance empirically. In 1866 he published a scientific paper in which he described these patterns of inheritance. Mendel had discovered genetics.

Lysenko convinced Stalin and other Communist Party leaders that organisms could be altered not only through their genetic inheritance, but also through environmental influences. According to his cock-and-bull story, exposure to cold, for example, would improve the genetics of wheat seed and lead to greater wheat harvests. He published scientific papers claiming that under the right environmental influences, wheat plants actually produced rye seed! This is like saying that if you raise dogs in the woods they'll give birth to foxes.

Crazy as it was, the idea appealed to Stalin. It conformed to and flattered party ideology, just as biblical creationism is given equal weight with Mendelian genetics in the curricula of some states of the USA because, although it is just as silly as Lysenko's theories of evolution, it conforms to party theocratic ideology.

Lysenko flourished and became President of the Lenin Academy of Agricultural Sciences. In 1938 he had millions of hectares of land planted with seed exposed to low temperature, the condition he had 'proven' would improve the genetics of the plant. When the grain failed to sprout, rather than blaming himself, he had the farmers charged with sabotage. Millions died from starvation and Soviet biology was irredeemably blighted for generations. While the rest of the world developed the new science of genetics, Russia stood still, not unlike

91

what could happen in the United States today if human embryo stem cell research continues to be prohibited for political reasons.

Lysenko had another ace up his sleeve. This Hero of the USSR, this recipient of the Order of Lenin and two Stalin prizes, this flimflam man, convinced Stalin that his theory of genetics applied to people too. Environmental influences, he continued to preach, affect heredity, so if you raise people in a Communist environment in which they are taught the precepts of Communism and then breed from them, they will give birth to baby Communists. That would take a long time to prove so to confirm his theory he used dogs. The breed that is today called the Black Russian terrier, was developed at the Soviet Red Star Army Kennels to prove Lysenko's theories.

World War Two interrupted Lysenko's breeding programme, so it wasn't until 1952 that significant numbers of dogs—initially crosses of giant schnauzers, Airedales and Rottweilers but eventually involving up to 20 breeds—were produced. These giant dogs were trained to attack, then bred to produce a new generation that had 'inherited their parents' learning' and also naturally attacked. The fact that the dogs in the breeding programme were selected for their genetic aggression potential was disregarded. The 'Black Russian terrier' became the Red Army's favourite canine.

Until 1990, the breed was rarely seen outside the old Soviet Empire but when the Iron Curtain collapsed, Black Russian terriers started appearing both legally and illegally, especially in Finland and in Sweden, where they've now had a formal name change to '*Svart*' or Black terrier. Their communist ancestry has been tactfully forgotten.

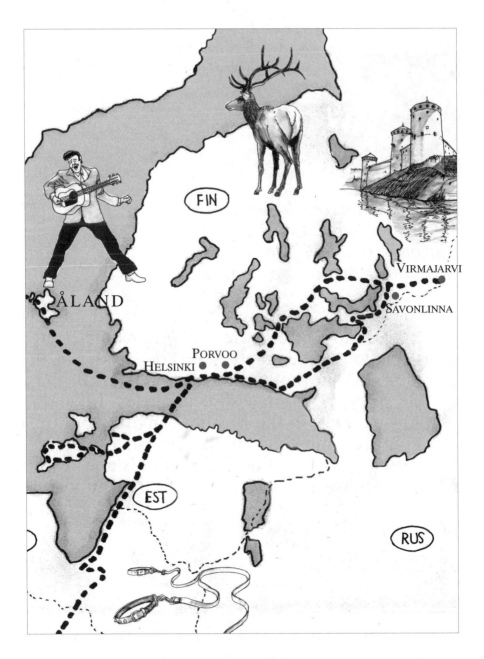

CHAPTER THREE

FINLAND

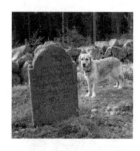

FINLAND

People per square kilometre	*15*
Dogs per square kilometre	*1.5*
Lingonberries per hectare	*6 tons*
Elvis impersonators on Åland	*1*

Side by side on a sloping hillside covered in grey-green deer moss and scarlet red lingonberries, in a forest glade on the small island of Prästo, in the Åland islands in the heart of the Gulf of Bothnia are old Muslim and Jewish cemeteries. I couldn't find any carvings in the Muslim cemetery but on a red granite tombstone in the Jewish cemetery I made out the date, 1831. The Åland islands which sit between Sweden and Finland are a quirky and unique oddity, but these ancient burial grounds were quite unexpected.

*   *   *

The duty-free shop on the three-hour ferry from Kappelskär north of Stockholm, to Åland's main town Mariehamn, was a clue to that uniqueness. Åland is a province of Finland and has the euro as currency, but duty free survives here, even though it's been abolished between all other countries in the EU. Åland has its own flag, its own pale-blue-on-white licence plates for its cars and its own stamps. There are fewer than 26,000 Ålanders but they hope to become the most influential minority in the EU.

The Åland guidebook I picked up on the ferry was an insight into the cultural scene on the islands. Ronald Karlsson, the local Elvis impersonator was singing at the Eckero Hotel, renamed GraceÅland for his appearances. 'He sounds like Elvis, he moves like Elvis. Ronald Karlsson has got it!' the guide effused. Other ads asked me to try the native apple liqueur, *'Ålvados'* or taste the cheeses, *'Stormskar'* and *'Bomarsund'*.

The ferry journey was amazingly cheap at 75 Swedish kronor—that's around six pounds—for me, my dog and my 6 metre long Roadtrek, but my fellow passengers were a different ilk to the sophisticated Swedes who used the Gotland ferry. These dour sourpusses were on a round trip booze cruise, devoting a day to stocking up on tax-free alcohol. The 75 kronor was their ticket of admission to the duty-free shop.

*   *   *

On Åland, all was still green. The moderating effect of the surrounding seas meant there had not yet been freezing nights on the islands, although on mainland Sweden some trees had already been touched by frost—yellow-leafed birches, red-leafed maples.

Four paved highways, 1, 2, 3 and 4, cover the compass directions out of Mariehamn.

Highway 3 led south to a ferry to the island of Föglö and I fancied being a Fogle on Föglö but in the end I decided to head north on Highway 2 towards Prästo where there was a large nature reserve. About half an hour out of Mariehamn I turned off the dire sub-Eurovision Song Contest music on the radio, and off the main highway as well, on to a mute red-coloured, empty, gravelled side-road. I parked by a wide inlet from the bay and took Macy for a walk past meadows white with marguerites, then past a row of red-painted fishermen's cottages into sun-dappled deciduous woods of ash, oak and elm. An Arctic hare with a grey-brown summer coat hadn't noticed my dog's approach, and Macy shot off in pursuit, deep into the forest. I lost her for half an hour. She re-emerged just as I was asking the only person I met, a local fisherman returning from further up the inlet, if he had seen her.

'The dogs come back when they are tired. They smell the fish,' he explained, mysteriously, as there were no fish.

Swedish is the spoken language of Åland, the only official language. In fact, although this is part of Finland, the Finnish language is not officially recognised here. Åland should logically be part of Sweden but because of the Russians it isn't. Geographically, it's much closer to Sweden, only 45 kilometres off the coast, and like Öland it was once a vast royal hunting park for Swedish kings. Culturally it is thoroughly Swedish too, although curiously, the Swedish fisherman I was speaking to didn't look prototypically Swedish. He had a scraggly dark moustache, dark straight hair, a broad nose and hazel eyes.

'Caught any fish?' I asked.

'No,' he succinctly replied, then after a pause he

added, 'Not yet.'

'What do you fish for?'

'*Gadd*. They come back now, from deep water. Here,' and he turned his head towards the waters of the inlet.

'You need a fishing permit,' he continued, somewhat sternly, assuming I was here to fish and as he told me this he took a packet labelled 'Kicks' from his fishing jacket and placed a small wrapped condom in his mouth.

It's times like this when you need to make an instant decision. Do you tell the guy he just made a howler of a mistake, or do you just act casual and cool and assume he wants to protect his tongue? Then, remembering something about my classmates from the prairies back in my university days in Canada I asked another question, 'Was that a pouch of chewing tobacco?'

'Yes. *Snus*,' he replied and he paused once more before continuing.

'This is how we make Finland leave the EU.'

I asked what he meant.

'*Snus* is legal in Sweden but it is banned everywhere. We have our own laws in Åland. It is legal here. The EU fine us for selling it. We want to tell the court why we sell it but they do not listen to us because we are not a country. We are part of Finland.'

'So?' I asked.

'In Åland we are responsible for our health. We make our own laws. Next year, when Finland is president of the EU we do not accept the EU constitution. We have a treaty with Finland. If we do not accept the constitution, Finland cannot accept it. There will be no EU constitution because the EU interrupt our affairs.'

He paused once more but now he was on a veritable roll.

'It is not just about *snus*. We shoot ducks in the spring but the EU tell us it is forbidden. My father fishes with nets but he is told it is not allowed. We make a mistake when we vote to join the EU but now we correct it. Brussels is too far away. The EU is shit.'

*   *   *

The coniferous woodlands at Prästo were blanketed in blueberries and lingonberries. I decided to disregard Macy's earlier misdemeanour and let her go where her nose took her, but in this setting of lichen-covered red granite and unending stretches of spongy pale green-white deer-moss she was always in sight. By an array of old decaying tree stumps I come upon a battalion of porcini mushrooms like a collection of champagne corks, and collected some for supper. At a height of land I climbed a watchtower from where I could see an arc of still, blue waters beyond the forests. It was while descending to the west from the watchtower and heading towards open water that I chanced upon the Muslim and Jewish cemeteries.

I would have missed them but for a sign reading *'Gravplatser'* on which there was a star of David and a crescent curling around a small star. I couldn't discern individual graves in the Muslim cemetery. There was nothing but lingonberry ground cover surrounding pink granite rocks with their quartz and black mica minerals reflecting sparkles of late afternoon light.

100

The adjacent Jewish cemetery, also surrounded by a rectangular wall of rough-hewn granite boulders and rocks, seemed well tended. The gravestones were all upright and although the Hebrew engravings were almost illegible on most, there was one stone—the one with the year 1831, that had been cleaned of its lichen, revealing the lettering on both sides. It was the grave of a man named '*Naftali*'.

Small pebbles had been placed on the top of each stone very recently, an old Jewish tradition. While forest flies hovered in the soft shafts of sunlight in the woods I picked some lingonberries and sitting in the stillness, looking through the dappled birch trees to the sparkling water beyond, watching dragonflies dart languidly in the air, I thought that this is the type of place, nourishing forest berries, that I'd like to be buried.

*   *   *

Now that I was aware of the small brown signposts like the one that had lead me to the graveyards, I noticed others and followed them east for around a mile, over the rocky hill to other cemeteries, Lutheran and Roman Catholic but also Greek Orthodox and Russian Orthodox.

On the island of Åland itself, just before the bridge to Prästo, stand the remains of a great Russian fort, Bomarsund, which the British and French forces destroyed in 1854 during the Crimean War. It marked the most westerly outpost of the far-flung Russian Empire. The main road goes straight through what was once the heart of the fort.

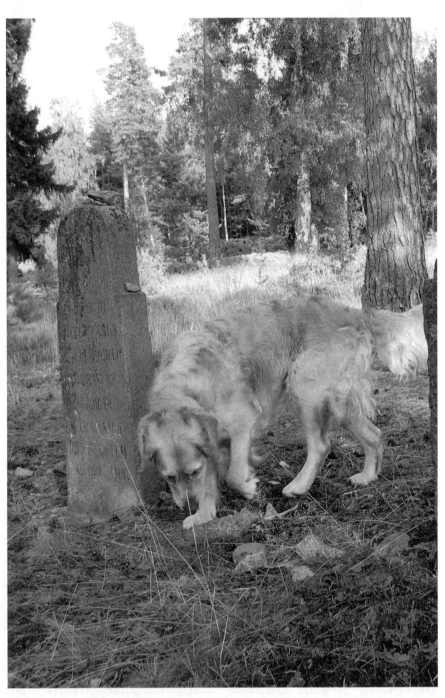

JEWISH GRAVES AT A CEMETERY HIDDEN IN THE WOODS AT PRÄSTO

Åland was a forgotten part of the 'Great Game' played by the Turkish, French, British and Russian empires. For millennia, both Åland and Finland had been part of Sweden but in 1807, to punish the Swedes for siding with the British, Napoleon Bonaparte 'gave' Finland and Åland to Russia, a demonstration of his authority as Europe's *de facto* ruler.

Thousands of Russian troops moved in and, soon after, plans were made to build a great fort at Bomarsund. The Muslim and Jewish burial grounds contain the graves of Russia's conscript soldiers who were engaged in preparing the grounds for this fort. These and a nearby Russian Orthodox burial ground were the first cemeteries. The burial grounds I visited later, on the east side of the island, were not prepared until the late 1840s. For decades thousands of Russian troops occupied the islands and some married, or for that matter raped, local girls. That's probably why the Ålander I met did not look distinctively Swedish, or Finnish for that matter.

The Crimean War was an epochal event in the continuing civil war between east and west Europe. It may be named after the location of the greatest battles, in what is now the Ukraine, but the Crimean War took place here too, in the far north.

British leaders feared the Russians would encroach on Afghanistan and India. Using the pretext of protecting Catholics and Catholic possessions in the Ottoman Empire (the Ottoman Sultan had recognised by treaty that Russia was the protector of Orthodox Christians living in the Ottoman Empire, and France the protector of Roman Catholics), a joint force of British, French,

103

Turkish and Sardinian troops attacked the Russian troops that had invaded Ottoman territories in what is now Moldova and Romania. To prevent Russia's Baltic fleet from reaching that theatre of war, the Baltic was blockaded by a combined force of British and French fleets.

The fort at Bomersand was destroyed but Åland remained in Russian hands until the end of World War One, when Finland achieved independence from Russia. The Ålanders petitioned to join Sweden, the Finns refused and Britain sought a compromise by referring the 'Åland Question' to the new League of Nations. They decided that Åland should remain part of new Finland but the islands should be permanently demilitarised and have their culture—including their use of the Swedish language—protected by law.

That evening I camped out in front of the remains of Bomarsund. While there was still light we walked east over the smooth coastal granite shoreline. I picked a bagful of orange sea buckthorn berries, cursing each time I pricked my fingers on the sharp thorns that protected the fruit. Tufts of violet and white flowers grew from cracks in the granite, purple loosestrife, wild chives and sea mayweed.

Macy cavorted among the reeds that surrounded the glistening rocks in the shallows of the still water. British and Russian cannon balls had flown directly over where she was now standing. One of those cannon balls landed on the British ship *Helca* and midshipman Charles David Lucas seized the ball and tossed it overboard, where it exploded harmlessly. He was awarded the first ever Victoria Cross. Two more would be

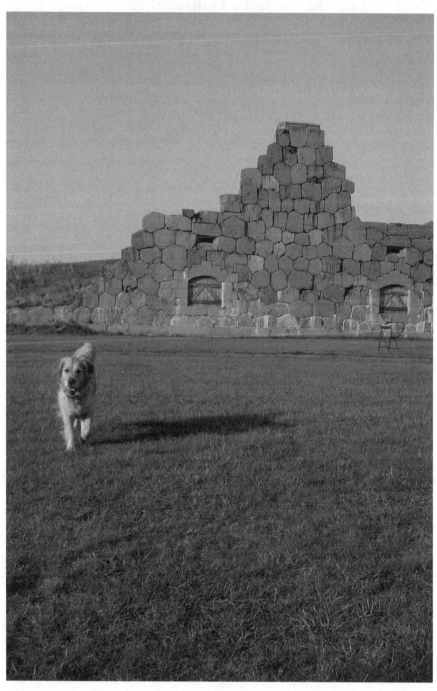

THE REMAINS OF BOMARSUND, THE RUSSIAN FORT
ON THE WAY TO PRÄSTO

awarded at the battle of Bomarsund.

An excellent Åland meal
Chop and fry porcini mushrooms in unsalted Swedish butter.
Microwave a Danish potato. Open it and fill it with butter and a sprinkling of crispy, fried Danish onions.
Add a whole smoked Gotland flounder.
Sit on a chair in front of the massive granite blocks of a Russian fort with your dog lying by your side and as a majestic sea eagle floats above in the sky, watch the sun set as you eat.
Finish the meal with a bowl of fresh picked, tart, sea buckthorn berries.

Night descended swiftly and with the darkness came the mosquitoes so we retreated into the Roadtrek. Tove Jansson, in her life-affirming novel *Sommerboken—The Summer Book*, wrote about her childhood summers in the archipelago to the east of the Åland islands: 'Each year, the bright Scandinavian summer nights fade away without anyone's noticing. One evening in August you have an errand outdoors, and all of a sudden it's pitch black. A great, warm, dark silence surrounds the house. It is still summer, but the summer is no longer alive. It has come to a standstill; nothing withers, and autumn is not ready to begin.'

That's how it was on Åland that night.

*   *   *

I spent the next four days in mainland Finland but not once after talking to the Swedish-speaking

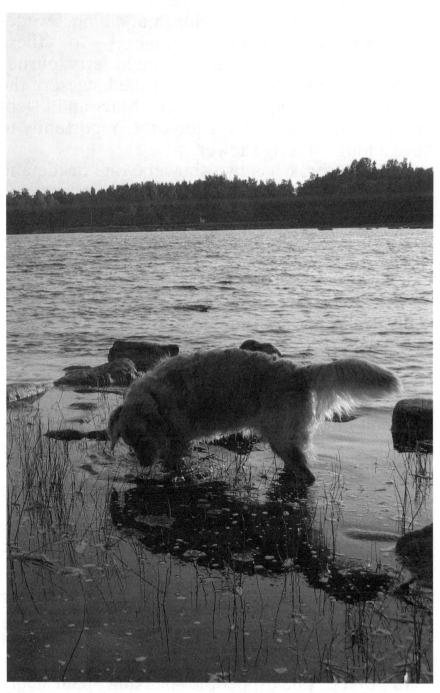

MACY CAVORTED AMONG THE REEDS

Ålander did I manage to get more than a few words in response from a phlegmatic Finn. Swedes are positively manic compared to these expressionless people. The overnight ferry journey from Mariehamn to Helsinki was the longest of the 10 boat trips yet, almost 10 hours. Macy and I slept in a starboard cabin and I took the opportunity to have a long relaxing shower.

The Roadtrek has two showers, one inside and one outside but after trying the inside one and accidentally washing my bed I decided to stick to campsite showers. I hadn't stayed in a campsite since Denmark. I'd planned to take the ferry to Turku and visit Muumimaailma—Moomin World—a theme park based on Tove Jansson's whimsical characters but that ferry was fully booked so Macy was holding her bladder for a longer journey.

The weather was holding perfectly too—another cloudless, fresh day. By the time we got to Helsinki at 10 a.m. it was already 23°C. The ferry dock is close to the Finnish President's residence in the centre of understated Helsinki and an official visit from the Tanzanian President delayed our exit from the city but permitted Macy to sit, wag and salute as the visiting dignitary reviewed the honour guard that had been mustered for his arrival. We headed east towards the Russian border and St. Petersburg just beyond, stopping for breakfast in a harvested field, surrounded by white butterflies and massive, green fluorescent damselflies.

In Porvoo, I heard people speaking Spanish and it sounded so friendly, so familiar, so warm, that I spontaneously found myself saying '*Hola*' to them.

They responded with smiles and chatter and looked endearingly relaxed and approachable compared to the dour Finns. Old Porvoo is certainly attractive—a classic grid of cobbled streets and alleyways lined with pastel-painted wooden homes and shops. It looks very Swedish for that's just what it was: the Swedish city of Børga.

Macy loved it in Porvoo. She got incessantly stroked by tourists, Spanish, Japanese, American; Porvoo is that type of place. Seeing a heart-stoppingly attractive raven-haired Russian mum perked me up and I asked, through sign language, whether I could take a photo of Macy with her and her family of three gorgeous children. She smiled and took my camera and took photos of Macy with me and her kids instead. The square-faced locals avoided eye contact. We rambled along the river, opposite the *Falu* red, riverside warehouses, and had a coffee at a café amongst the craft boutiques, where Macy was neither acknowledged nor offered water by my waitress, as I had now come to expect.

*　　　*　　　*

Highway E18 is the route to Russia. You can feel through the ride it gives that this road suffers the expansions and contractions of annual freezes and thaws. The landscape was as monotonous and boring as the Finns themselves, flatter than the prairies, yet my map said that this was a scenic route. Fortunately the road signs were bilingual and I read the Swedish as if it were my mother tongue.

At Strömfors, where there's an interesting

octagonal church, I stopped for an hour and chanced on a magnificent wild raspberry bush by the mill stream. Dessert. At Kotka, the bilingual road signs ended. Official signs were now only in Finnish although billboards were in Russian as well as Finnish. It took a lot of concentration on my part to figure out that Pietari was Finnish for St. Petersburg.

Near the border I stopped at a market selling industrial-size packages of Fairy Liquid, Arial and Pedigree Chum dog food and massive tins of olives, engine oil and coffee to returning Russians. Just before the border crossing, where a kilometre-long convoy of trucks waited to get processed through customs inspection into Russia, I turned north on to the 'Via Karelia', an even more boring road—if that's possible—through land devoid of all character.

Interspersed amongst the spindly and insignificant trees were occasional tired-looking homes and a few harvested fields. The most impressive thing about the rest area where I stopped to give Macy a walk was the sheer quantity of toilet paper strewn about—Olympian in quantity compared to the similar site I'd chanced upon in northern Germany. Everywhere there were thundering Russian logging trucks, black fumes belching from their diesel stacks.

Near Savonlinna I turned off the main road looking for a suitable campsite and drove for over 10 kilometres along a meandering tree-lined elevation, an unexpected, natural causeway through water—an Ice Age esker. There was a hotel at the end of the causeway with electricity points in its parking lot and I thought these might

110

be for motorhomes, but they were for winter block heaters, not for overnight camping. I was told I couldn't stay and moving on, found a dirt road by a lake. I parked where the road ended beyond a series of summer cottages, let Macy out, then fired up the generator, plugged in my laptop and in the early evening light started catching up on writing. Around an hour later, a Finn motorcycled up, stopped and stared. He didn't get off his bike.

'*Hei,*' I acknowledged in the local tongue. He stared back impassively.

'Got a ball?' Macy asked with her eyes.

Nothing. Eventually, without expression, without moving his lips, he spoke.

'What are you doing?'

'I'm writing about driving through Finland and about how accommodating and wonderful the people are.'

There was a pause. It took a minute for him to collect his thoughts.

'I live here,' he replied

'You lucky guy,' I responded, but he didn't do irony.

'You will not stay here,' he said

There was no inflection to his voice so I couldn't tell whether he was making a statement or asking a question, but either way I hightailed it out of there just as soon as he and his farting little bike departed.

*   *   *

The sound of the wind through the birch leaves that night was like the roar of breakers on a Pacific shore. It had rained heavily and by serendipity

111

rather than planning I'd ended up finding a perfect wood to camp in. I didn't know until we went walkabout that I was in woods planted by the Finnish Forest Research Institute at Punkaharju. That morning hike became a private lesson in tree ecology.

A stand of cedars looked extraordinarily familiar to me, just like the cedars at our summer cottage in Ontario. They were Ontario cedars, *Thuja occidentalis*, planted here by the research institute to see how they fared 15° farther north than their Canadian home. Further on was a grove of Korean cedar with brilliant green leaves that were almost white underneath. Beside that was a paper birch grove; these trees grow mixed with black spruce in Ontario, in boggy, poorly drained soil, but they didn't seem to be thriving here.

In the birch grove behind the Roadtrek falling seeds were being collected in upturned umbrella-like containers throughout the plantation. The western cedars weren't looking too good either but the Douglas fir from British Columbia were thriving. Near them were Siberian stone pines, lamp-post straight with high crowns. The sign said they provided nourishment for people in time of famine, and animal fodder too.

Paper-thin, ochre-coloured bark was peeling from the *Pinus silvestris* trees and further beyond were 15 different varieties of *Picea abies*—seven from Finland, five from the old Soviet Union and three from Central Europe. Each was marked by the latitude and longitude of its origin: Finland 63°, 5 minutes latitude, 29°, 50 minutes longitude; Romania 47°, 20 minutes latitude, 25°, 21 minutes longitude; Belgium 48°, 4 minutes latitude, 6°,

53 minutes longitude. I was wandering through the future of planned forestry in Finland.

*   *   *

The road to Savonlinna was as straight as the plantation pines, and once more elevated above the surrounding land—probably for good drainage. At school bus-stops little kids were playing with their Game Boys and the older kids had earphones in their ears. No one made eye contact with anyone. The rain had been refreshing but it powerfully reinvigorated the mosquitoes and those bloodsuckers' bites on the back of my neck were really bugging me.

In Savonlinna I parked and walked with Macy. Everyone averted their eyes when I gave a *'Hei!'* greeting, so much so I wondered whether I was really saying 'Hello' or unwittingly telling them to 'Piss off'. Was I putting the wrong emphasis, somehow, on the word? I saw a Samoyed. I'd read that the Finno-Ugrian languages include Estonian and Samoyed so I said *'Hei!'* to the dog but he didn't respond either.

Medieval Olavinlinna Castle in Savonlinna is a show-stopper. Olavinlinna Castle was built over 500 years ago by the Swedes to protect the eastern flank of their empire. More often than not, however, the owner-occupiers were Russians. In the 1920s, original drawings of the proposed Russian fortifications at Bomarsund on Åland were discovered here. The Savonlinna Opera Festival held each July inside the castle, must be magnificent.

As I walked along the waterside park looking at

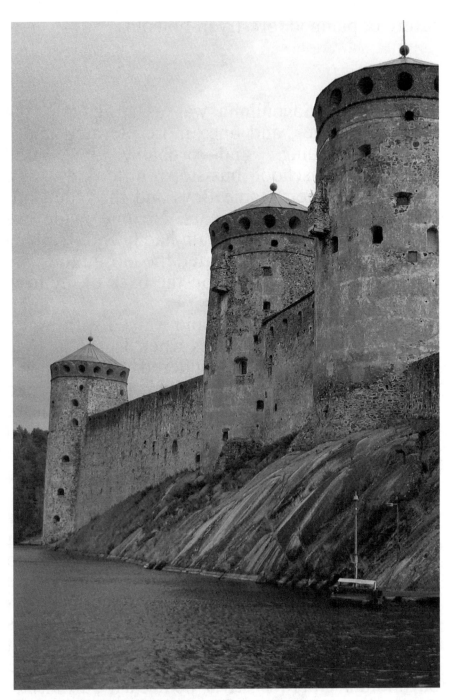

OLAVINLINNA CASTLE IN SAVONLINNA

this brooding island fortress a very, very, long black logging boat from St. Petersburg with peeling paint passed through the narrow channel between the shoreline and the castle. A footbridge to the castle had been opened to allow the boat to squeeze through.

Macy entertained herself by eyeing the local ducks while I looked in the windows of the tourist shops. They featured Sami kitsch and Sami art, much as Canadian tourist shops feature Inuit art. Devoid of anything unique within their own dominant cultures, both Canada and Finland borrow the traditions of their indigenous minorities in an attempt to create a unique national identity.

We spent another hour walking in blustery wind along the rocky shores of the lake. Savonlinna is obviously a hub for lake traffic, and we passed two old wooden church longboats amongst the reeds on the shore, past moored vintage lake-steamers and other dog walkers. I hand signalled 'hellos' to the locals but as far as these po-faced people were concerned, the tourist season was now over and they could return to their natural gloomy personalities.

I gave up and left and with Barry the Australian Sat Nav guy giving instructions, I headed for the most easterly point in the European Union for no better reason than to say I'd been there, stopping at Kerimaki for Macy to roll on the grounds of the largest wooden church in the world. It was built in 1847, seats over 3000 and was locked. We drove on.

Barry took me onto a potholed dirt road south of Joensuu where gravel had been sent cascading

115

on to the road by torrential rain. Australian though he was, he successfully directed me on to highway 494, then 495 to Ilomantsi then 496 and finally 74. I was alone in the heart of Karelia and I think I was falling in love with Barry.

It was overcast and cool, in the low 10°s. The roadside verges had been cut recently and snow poles had been placed to guide trucks for winter snow ploughing. The land looked forlorn and it was difficult for me to comprehend that war has been its major product. In my lifetime this has been a land of refugees and wintry death.

Karelia is the emotional heart of Finland, the inspiration for their national epic the Kalevala. For hundreds of years it has been a land of contention and shifting borders, fought over by the Swedish and Russian empires. By the early 1800s it was firmly within the Russian Empire, the eastern rim of the Russian-owned Grand Duchy of Finland. Karelia was the homeland of Finland's independence movement and with the collapse of Tsarist Russia, it became the proud heart, in 1920, of independent Finland.

Karelia's freedom was short lived. In the Winter War of 1939–1940, Stalin's Soviet troops invaded. Hundreds of thousands of Finnish Karelians were displaced but when Finland's David halted Stalin's Goliath, many were able to return to the homes. Not for long. In the Continuation War of 1941–1944, the Soviet Union permanently occupied much of Karelia. Hundreds of thousands of Karelians were displaced once more. The bisected Karelian culture has never recovered and now the land looks spent.

In Hattuvaara I stopped at the *'Taistelijan*

Talo'—the 'Fighter's House', a Winter War museum. The waitress at the museum café directed me to the nearby Frontier Guard Station where I was given a permit to drive to the Finnish-Russian border at Lake Virmajarvi, the most easterly point in the European Union. On the application form I applied 'yes' 'for a camera' and 'no' 'for a weapon'. The impassive, green-uniformed Frontier Guard actually made eye contact with me, spoke English and acknowledged Macy's presence with a nod and almost a smile so I took the opportunity to squeeze a few words out of him.

He was a local guy from Naarva, a short distance further north, and had worked in the North Karelia Frontier Guard District for three years. Most of his time was spent on surveillance work to prevent smuggling but each spring his detachment was responsible for cutting and clearing the border with Russia, for ensuring that yellow buoys in waterways were positioned correctly after the winter ice thawed, and for attaching yellow plastic markers to appropriate trees.

Sometimes their security dogs—German shepherds—accompanied them but at home he had a *Karjalankarhukoira*, a Karelian bear dog. I knew about these impressive black-and-white hunting dogs and asked if he hunted with his. He didn't but others in his village used theirs for elk hunting. Two litters of pups had been born that summer to neighbours' bear dogs. They were outdoor dogs that survived the winters well in their dog houses.

What a terrific name, 'bear dog'. If you're called

a 'bear dog' I bet you automatically get respect from other dogs. You've got dignity, you've got stature. Compare that to being called a 'Nova Scotia duck-tolling retriever'. Karelian hunters really did use these dogs to hunt bear and, according to the Frontier Guard, some still do.

After the Winter War between Finland and Russia in 1939–40, Finland was compelled to give a large part of Karelia to Russia, the area that is today the Karelian Republic of Russia, and they created a new name for bear dogs on their side of the new border: Russo-European laikas. Genetically identical, this breed has now been bred to be a little larger than bear dogs on the Finnish side but they are used for the same purpose, to track silently, and when game is sighted to bark continuously. 'They are good watchdogs, very fierce,' I was told and I asked if any were used by the Frontier Guards for security. 'No. They are too not tame, too fierce.'

*   *   *

The most easterly point in the European Union is an open landscape of birch and pine trees in a virtual sea of carmine-coloured lingonberries. From the main highway, it's around 15 kilometres along dirt roads to the frontier. The most prominent of the rocks protruding from the road's surface have been painted red by Frontier Guards, to protect car chassis. At the end of the road we walked along a boardwalk in a restricted area marked by blue ropes to a platform overlooking Virmajarvi, Lake Virma.

This was the most northerly as well as the most

118

easterly point of my travels, 300 kilometres east of Istanbul, 70 kilometres east of St. Petersburg, 150 kilometres north of Anchorage, Alaska. This remote landscape, even under threatening skies was alluring and sublimely peaceful and while Macy contented herself by investigating the forest floor for life forms I got a Ziploc plastic bag and started picking lingonberries.

The lingonberry is the true fruit of the boreal forest. In Scandinavia I've seen it used for juice, sauce, preserves, jelly, syrup, ice cream, wine and liqueur. It probably has more English names than any other forest fruit: cowberry, moss cranberry, mountain cranberry, partridgeberry, red whortleberry, alpine cranberry or simply lingon or lingen.

Its shiny, leathery, dark green, evergreen leaves add vibrancy to the forest floor. At this time of year, when crops are abundant, the berries, or to be accurate the flower's ovaries, are so scarlet that the ground is as crimson as it is green. The plants, on their almost woody stems, stood proud above the surrounding moss and twig litter. In less than an hour I'd picked over three kilos, six to ten berries at a time off the tip of each branch.

The Swedes estimate there is an average of six tons of berries per hectare of forest, a massive natural harvest. Few people visit here because of the requirement for a permit but even so this sandy acidic soil looked like it produced twice the average harvest. I'd got permission at the 'Fighter's House' museum to stay overnight at the nearby *'Karhunkämmen'*, or 'Bear's Paw Cabin' and an inviting smell of wood-smoke poured out the door as I opened it.

Inside there was unlimited cut firewood and although it was only mid-afternoon I didn't want to prop the cabin door open and let mosquitoes in so I kindled a fire in the stone fireplace and lit the candles that a previous occupant had left, and that was all the light we needed. As long as I stayed outdoors Macy worked the reeds on the stony shore of the lake, raising ducks. When I retreated into the cabin's wonderland, she was soon at the door barking to come in too. The fireplace was also the stove and worked well enough for me to cook my supper.

BOILED LINGONBERRIES ON BUTTERED PENNE
Over a wooden fire, boil 200g of fresh picked lingonberries with an almost equal amount of sugar. No water is necessary. Set aside.
In water collected from a Finnish lake, boil Marks & Spencer penne until soft. Drain in a pasta strainer purchased from IKEA in Älmhult, then add 50g of butter and a pinch of salt. Stir well and pour the buttery pasta on to a plate.
Top with lingonberry sauce, sprinkle with pepper and eat to the light of a log fire.
Trust me. It works.

It was a two-day drive back to Helsinki and the ferry I'd take to Estonia. I learned that on dirt roads with a surface like a washboard, 40 mph was the optimum speed to avoid feeling every bump. Occasionally Barry the Sat Nav guy told me I was on an 'unnamed road', but he remained accurate wherever I travelled.

Winter firewood was stacked at every home. On a typically straight stretch of road I chanced upon

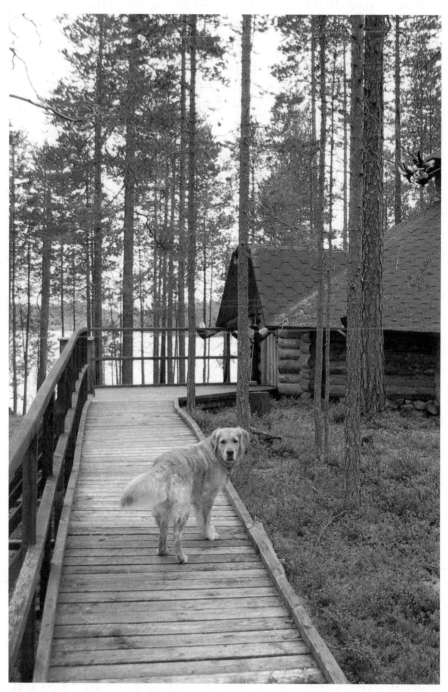

THE 'KARHUNKÄMMEN', OR 'BEAR'S PAW CABIN'
AT VIRMAJARVI

some local agriculture, a field of grazing Ayrshire cattle. I saw more Ayrshires than all other breeds combined while in Finland. In the next field were four cranes pecking through the cropped stubble, so I pulled off the road but as I did they stopped, looked at me and immediately took flight. That was the day's excitement.

Soon afterwards it began to rain and continued to pour torrentially until the evening. At an afternoon Macy-stop on a secondary logging road there were deer tracks so fresh they must have been made minutes before we arrived, but the rain convinced me to curtail the walk and just keep on driving. I camped that night by a bog in the woods and listened to the mosquitoes throwing themselves against the screens. I killed plenty in the Roadtrek the following day, all blood-filled and wondered whether it was Macy's or mine.

Four hours out of Helsinki I stopped to examine some road kill. It was a racoon dog and its hind legs, but not its pelvis, had been crushed. Pancaked. After its legs were run over, it had dragged itself to the shoulder of the road. I could see the scratch marks where its clenched front claws had dug deep in the gravelly dirt. There it had died, very recently, from clinical shock.

This female was young, born in the spring. Her teeth, less blade-like than a dog's or a fox's, were Hollywood white and her brindle black and fawn-brown body hair was shiny and healthy. Her feet and face mask were the colour of a black bear. She probably weighed around six or seven kilograms—about the same as a lean Cavalier King Charles Spaniel.

I'd never seen a racoon dog before but knew

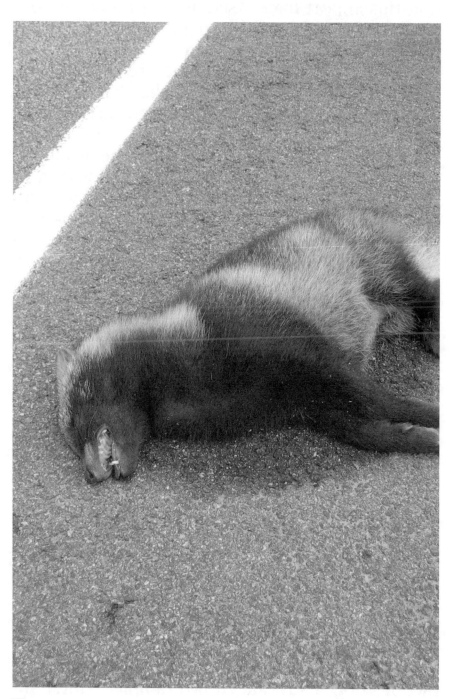

THE RACOON DOG, NEITHER RACOON NOR DOG

that this import from Asia, neither a racoon nor a 'dog', had found itself a perfect ecological niche in Finland. I had passed at least 20 racoon dog road kills just south of Varkaus, before I stopped to look at this one. In Russia and the Baltic States it is, along with the red fox, the prime carrier of the rabies virus.

The racoon dog arrived in Europe when the Soviets imported them into Belarus and Russia for fur farming. Some were released into the wild not far from the Finnish border and by the mid-1970s they were expanding their range by on average 40 kilometres a year, until they populated most of south and central Finland. They continue to spread inexorably westwards and southwards and have now got as far as eastern France, Switzerland and Austria.

Their numbers in Finland increased almost logarithmically. In 1970 Finnish hunters killed around 700. By 1990 over 70,000 were killed annually by hunters. Who knows how many are killed on Finland's roads where the animal's unique behaviour makes it particularly susceptible to injury and death.

There are now more racoon dogs than red foxes in Finland but they, as well as badgers, seem to accommodate to each other. As omnivores they all fill the same ecological niche, but while foxes prefer small mammals such as voles, and badgers selectively eat invertebrates such as snails, racoon dogs prefer plant material—especially berries.

Judging from her plumpness the road-kill racoon dog had laid down ample winter fat reserves by gorging on lingonberries. If these or blueberries aren't available the raccoon dogs are very adaptable and willingly live near people's homes, living off our refuse. I was surprised at first by how short and delicate her legs were. Her paws were much smaller than a cat's, thin and dainty.

While the black mask of facial hair makes this animal look strikingly similar to a racoon, it's not a relation. It's a true member of the canine family and like the fox it's a nocturnal woodland forager, working from sunrise to sunset. It uses selected toileting sites and survives the winter by sleeping through the snowy months, sometimes sharing a den with badgers. Badgers take to their dens earlier in the autumn and wake later in spring so they are probably unaware of snoozing racoon dogs sharing their dens.

The weak link in the racoon dog's coping strategies is its response to danger. Faced with mortal threat it feigns death. It drops on its side, motionless, with its tongue hanging out. Most predators respond to movement. Their instinct to chase, capture and kill is triggered by flight. The hunting instinct is muted by stillness unless the hunter is a car or a truck. When confronted by the threatening fiery eyes of headlights on a highway, rather than running to the far side of the road as a fox would do, the racoon dog drops where it is and plays dead. True death inevitably follows, sometimes a prolonged death as happened to the racoon dog I stopped to look at.

*   *   *

At a petrol station north of Helsinki, Marcus came over to admire the Roadtrek. At last, I'd met a pro-active Finn. He told me he wrote Garrison

125

Keillor-type books and was a Finnish Broadcasting TV producer. The trouble was, although I'd finally met a Finn who was willing to tell me his story, I didn't have time to listen. I had to catch the Seacat to Tallinn.

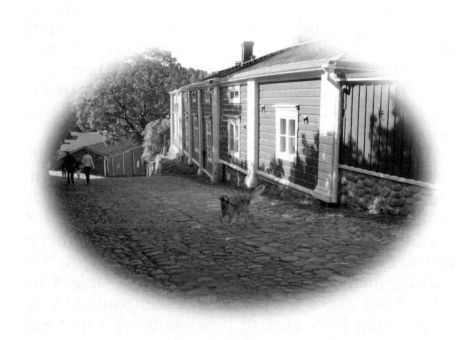

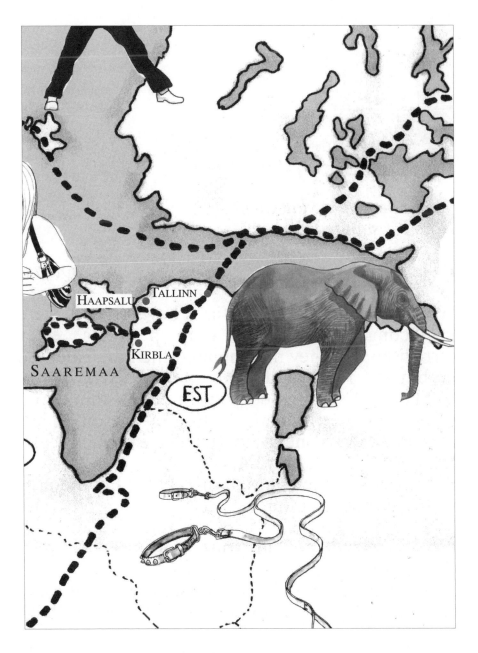

CHAPTER FOUR

ESTONIA

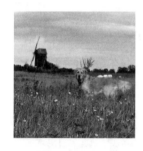

ESTONIA

People per square kilometre	*29*
Dogs per square kilometre	*3*
Elephants with both tusks extracted	*1*
Windmills on Saaremaa	*Quaint*

'They were gangsters! Mafia! They said they were protecting us but they were parasites. They terrorised us. They manipulated the law. Talented criminals. Rewarded with power. What they disliked was suppressed. You could not think. You could not be human. It was a prison. They appointed everyone, even the village councils. The State didn't exist, only the Party.'

The man looked at Macy and at his Labrador as they sniffed each other.

'Dogs were our substitute for real life. They did not know you could trust dogs. Speak your thoughts to them.'

'He is still angry,' his wife said apologetically. 'He must learn to get on with life and not just look back.'

Welcome to the former Soviet Union. To Estonia. I was entering the region where, between 1914 and 1945 Europe took leave of its senses, the perimeter of the most recent battleground between Germany and Russia in Europe's ongoing civil war.

My angry friend was waiting with his yellow Labrador and his wife for the ferry to Saaremaa, a large Baltic island that Estonians say still holds the true heart of the country, but by the time I met him I had already been primed about life during the Soviet era.

*   *   *

A few days beforehand I'd taken the Seacat from Helsinki to Tallinn because it was the fastest route to Estonia, but when the voice on the intercom said, 'We recommend that you remain seated during your journey because of strong winds,' I knew that Macy would hate it. When I got back to the vehicle deck, two hours after I'd left her, she'd retreated to the pillows on the bed and was shivering relentlessly. She needed several minutes of tight squeezing for the shivering to diminish.

Estonian Customs minutely inspected the Roadtrek's registration documents and while they did so, I minutely inspected Macy and removed two more feeding ticks from both armpits. Judging from their size they'd been feeding for a day or two. I applied more Frontline. Just off the ferry I stopped at a Norwegian Statoil petrol station and tanked up on cheap petrol while local, jackbooted, black-garbed guys working for the Scandinavian security firm Falck patrolled the forecourt.

I parked and went on an afternoon walking tour of the Old Town but it was like Venice at chaotic carnival time, dozens of tour groups led by tour guides waving paddles with numbers on them. It was frenetic and, attractive as the town was, unpleasant. Estonia may be the new EU but a beer here was more expensive than one in Helsinki. Shop girls gave Macy cuddles and Russian words of affection while I inspected and bought bolts of white linen for Julia. Out on the cobbled streets tourists treated my dog with the same affection. 'Better than a wife,' an Italian tourist said to me in English after kissing Macy on the top of her head.

In the park outside the walls of the Old Town drunk Finns lurched along the paths. Old *babushkas* were begging from tourists outside the onion-domed ochre-and-white Russian Orthodox Church. After the emptiness of Sweden and Finland, I found the crowds disconcerting so I left town and headed south over land as flat as a Dutch *polder*, avoiding the stray dogs that wandered across the highway.

*　　　*　　　*

In Arto Paasilinna's masterpiece of a little novel *The Year of the Hare*, which the publisher calls 'a picaresque novel with an ecological theme', the Finnish anti-hero, Vatanen, is befriended by Police Superintendent Savolainen. The policeman is 'a youngish man, probably a recent graduate in jurisprudence, in the sticks as a stage in his career.' Vatanen rescues an injured hare and is invited to stay at Savolainen's fishing cabin and sauna beside a lake in the forest.

Around an hour and a half out of Tallinn I saw a hotel sign with a camping symbol, stopped for the night and met Ismo Savolainen, a Finnish university graduate who had given up his high-pressure banking job in Helsinki and moved with his partner to this new frontier of Estonia to buy and run a hotel and sauna. For the next few days each time I saw Ismo I could only see Superintendent Savolainen; they were both prototypical Finns, self-sufficient, independent, rural, and they both had a sauna and, of course, the same name.

*   *   *

It was a good move to stay there. The Ruunawere Hotell was an old coach house on the road from St. Petersburg to Riga, built in 1700. Not only did I get a campsite but for my 10 euros I also got my own sauna, shower, lounge, outdoor hot tub, garden table and conversation with the Savolainens. Ismo took me on a tour, proudly pointing out the old limestone floor and an impressive funnel of a chimney dating back to the 1500s, large enough to hang and smoke a couple of deer in. It's one of only a few such chimneys in the entire country, he explained.

The inn itself was on a meandering dirt road that parallels the new EU-funded main highway a few hundred metres to the east. The ancient meadows between the old and new roads had been burnt by a frost. Trees were reddened with autumn colours. Apple and crab apple trees flourished on the verges, as did flowering mint and bushes laden with tart, powder-blue, blackberries.

I learned from Ismo that these were in fact bearberries, 'karhunvatukka' in Finnish, 'karumarjad' in Estonian, 'björnbör' in Swedish. In Estonian they are also called 'poldmarad' or 'field berries'. Ismo explained that until the authorities

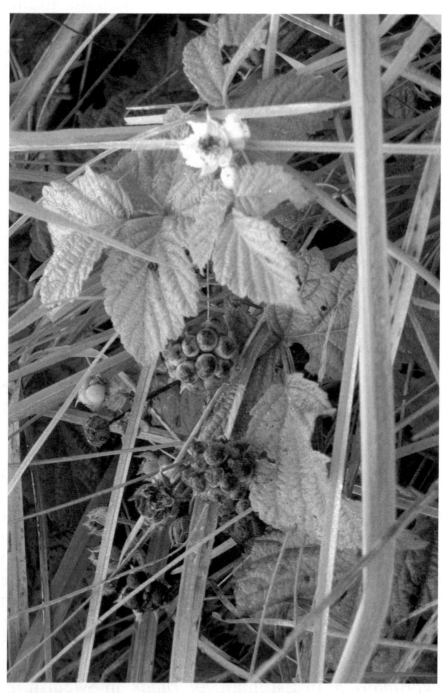

Bearberries, 'karumarjad' in Estonian

forced people to leave their farms in the 1950s to work on collective farms, there had been many houses along the road by the post station. All that was left of these were some stone foundations and those apple trees. I filled my pockets and later returned with bags to make serious collections.

Back at the inn Ismo explained that old inns existed every 30 kilometres along the ancient road, and were all of a similar style. An Estonian couple had bought the next one south and had come over to see how the Finns had restored theirs. The next one to the north was derelict and unoccupied. I asked Ismo, who had a degree in international economics, what it was like living in a country that had so recently been out of bounds. He explained that as the national currency, the kroon, was tied to the euro, the economy, for him at least, was secure. He dealt mostly in euros. Not so for older people. Ismo told me that their fixed incomes hadn't moved with inflation and many now depended on help from private organisations in Finland. The mentality of the older generation was that the state controlled and made all decisions. They found it difficult, if not impossible, to cope with the reality of capitalism and fending for themselves.

'It is a good place for Finnish people to retire to. The cost of living is very low and although Estonian vocabulary and grammar are different, Finnish people can understand some Estonian. Phrases no longer used in one language are still used in the other. A pension from Finland is very good here. I think retired Finnish people now make one per cent of the country's population.'

I asked Ismo if he saw many British tourists and

he raised the fingers of one hand.

'That many this year. We get Dutch tourists because there is a vintage car parts fair each summer that Dutch dealers come to.'

Over a couple of beers he explained he had learned to not rush in Estonia, to go with the flow when it came to services and supplies. He'd had no problems with bureaucrats or neighbours. In fact they had all been encouraging and wished him well.

*   *   *

I spent a day driving the back roads of western Estonia, getting a feel of the country. The old coaching road wriggles worm-like along first one side then the other of the new straight E road, which is marked with English language signs stating 'This road built with EU support'. I wondered why, considering the nature of European tourism, it was not also explained in German.

The road signs were excellent, identical to those in Finland, but here there were also frequent signs indicating the distance to the next internet access point. There were drunks with cider bottles everywhere, young and old, even on remote country roads. I still don't know why. A consequence of high unemployment post-independence? Or is it just part of the place's immutable culture.

Most of the wooden buildings I drove past in the countryside—and there weren't many of them—were not painted. Until the Soviet era these buildings were as plentiful as anywhere else around the Baltic, but they were destroyed either in the war or after it when agriculture was collectivised. Occasional old homes were painted a mustard yellow with dark brown around the doors and windows, a colour scheme I later learned was part of Estonian rural vernacular design. Mostly I drove past passionless, rectangular grey-brick buildings. Some were individual homes, some were flat-roofed two, four or eight-family dwellings and some were factories or warehouses.

In one village I saw old *babushkas* wearing kerchiefs over their hair and elderly men with flowing chin whiskers—Old Believers, remnants of a persecuted Russian Orthodox community that moved here to the fringes of the Empire hundreds of years ago in order to practise their religion as they wanted. Their church services are still conducted in Old Church Slavonic, rather than Russian or, needless to say, Estonian.

Mid-morning I stopped to turn around and return to a derelict collective farm I'd passed, to examine and measure the bricks, and was instantly confronted by two fierce, barking Caucasian Owtcharkas, 50-kilo brutes hurling themselves against a chain-link fence. They would have killed Macy in a second. I'm bigger so I'd have taken a fraction longer to polish off.

The collective farm buildings had been long stripped of everything other than the very bricks in the walls. These were big, 25 by 20 by 10 centimetres and I was struck by how sloppily they were laid. I looked at the quality of construction and thought it was built by 'who gives a shit' bricklayers but then it dawned on me that these buildings were saying something else. This was 'Fuck you!' bricklaying.

At Kirbla there was an official explanation to why there are so few wooden homes, a rusty metal sign with the words, '14-17/7/41 Kirbla—destroyed by Red Army'. It showed a map of the vicinity and the legend had a flame symbol to indicate 'Living houses burned down by Red Army'. There was a flame symbol over every single farmstead on the map. The Red Army had scorched the earth. It had extinguished local history and eventually replaced it with Soviet blocks where function was more important than form. 'Burn the nests,' Lenin said, 'and the birds will not come back.'

Beyond Kirbla, I arrived at the ferry terminal linking the mainland to the islands of Muhu and Saaremaa and on this warm, cloudless day Macy introduced herself to a Labrador and then me to the Lab's owner. It was while waiting for the ferry that his blood pressure soared as he told me about the Soviet era.

Saaremaa shares similarities with Öland and Gotland. It's also built upon limestone bedrock although less of that is visible here. There are occasional alvars but they are muted and insignificant compared to those on the Swedish islands. It's on the same East Atlantic flyway as the Swedish islands, so the reeds surrounding the causeway to the island were covered by a flotilla of thousands of barnacle geese and mute swans. The road sign as I left the causeway from the island of Muhu and reached Saaremaa itself warned of elk for the next 5 kilometres, but as I rounded the first bend in the road I was confronted by a lazy Holstein staring me down. It had escaped its tether and was playing chicken with the Latvian tour

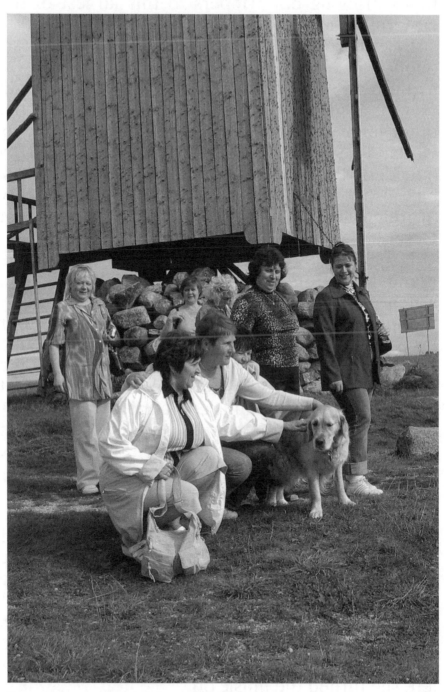

LATVIAN TOURISTS WITH MACY AT ANGLA

buses bringing day trippers to this largest of the eastern Baltic islands.

Elsewhere in this new country of needlessly duplicated vowels, ethnic Russians constitute over a quarter of the inhabitants but here on Saaremaa they now make up only one per cent. Like the other large Baltic islands—it's almost as large as Gotland—Saaremaa has been serially owned by outsiders, the usual Swedes, Danes and Russians, but also the Germans. For most of its history Saaremaa was a German fiefdom, the island of Oesel.

I spent two days casually driving around the island. My 1938 *L'Europe en Automobile* told me to watch out for the picturesque costumes worn by the inhabitants of Muhu but all the Latvian tour buses were heading for the 'working museum' village of Koguva on Muhu so I decided to give it a miss and forge ahead of them to the other tourist highlights—the windmills and a meteor crater. As on the mainland there were drunks in the most unexpected places, peeing by the roadside, staggering through villages. In the distance, deep-voiced dogs barked everywhere.

The five windmills that stand in a row at Angla are, in fact, serenely attractive. As Macy and I walked through the stillness around them, three Latvian tour buses arrived. The old lady in the tourist stand passionlessly turned on a CD of balalaika music and sat impassively once more, hoping that was enough to beguile the masses into parting with their kroons. As soon as the Latvians left, she turned the music off.

Kaali meteor crater was interesting too, until another pack of tour buses disgorged their day trippers. It's a water-filled basin in the middle of a mixed deciduous and coniferous woodland and over 100 metres wide. There's a steep climb to the rim of it, over earth thrown up by its impact around 700 BC.

Having ticked off the obligatory tourist destinations I took to the side-roads and walked away the first day, through juniper heath, pine forests, grasslands and stunning flowering meadows. We came across more windmills isolated in the middle of fields of poppy and cornflower and in the absence of tourists these were sublime. Back on the main roads, I headed for the most westerly point on the island, and it was good to see that the Soviet era functional, concrete-bunker bus-stops were being replaced by attractive pitch-roofed shelters made out of interlocking logs. I'd planned to stay the night at Loona Manor, an old manse that doubles as the Vislandi National Park Visitors' Centre and a hotel. It was closed but the parking lot provided me with a suitable camp ground and in late light I hiked with Mace along forest trails to the reed-lined sea shore and watched a flaming orange sun set over distant black, rocky islands.

ROADSIDE ESTONIAN DESSERT
Dice 200g of apples from abandoned Estonian apple trees and gently simmer in a touch of water and a little sugar until they are soft on the outside but still firm within.
Add 200g of fresh picked bearberries and heat them until they are hot but have not lost their shape.
With a scarf around your neck to keep you

*comfortable, sit outside and warm your stomach
with your tart Estonian dessert, wondering at the
beauty of a crisp Baltic night.*
*Employ a golden retriever for the occasion, to
act as your vigilant 'bear dog'.*

A crisp, cold night does wonders for eliminating
pesky mosquitoes and I spread the waterproof
seat-cover I used to protect the Roadtrek from
Macy's muddy paws over my own bed when I
started to freeze. For the first time in almost three
weeks I reached up and turned on the Roadtrek's
furnace before getting out of bed.

During the night I'd heard worryingly strange
shrieks in the distance, followed by intense dog
barking but that had stopped by dawn. I made
breakfast, apple and bearberry sauce on toasted
black bread, Bomarsund cheese from Åland and
black coffee, then headed for Kihelkonna and its
ancient harbour.

Seeing three cranes in the next field explained
the strident, sharp sounds I'd heard. This time I
managed to get some photos as they lofted into
graceful flight, their elongated necks pointing
toward the rising sun. The road to the harbour was
unimaginably beautiful in the sharp morning light,
a sparkling, rose-tinted, cobbled granite highway
almost two miles long through deciduous
woodland. It was straight out of a fairytale,
although neither on the drive to the harbour nor
back did I discover the right speed at which to
drive over large cobbles. Macy and I were both left
vibrating.

*   *   *

It was the stillest of mornings and the sea between me and the island of Vislandi to the west was a perfect mirror. The absolute silence was broken only by the barking and howling of dogs. They barked each time Macy or I moved. The harbour was used by local fishermen continuously from 1881 until 1940. After the war the Soviets destroyed the old fishing co-operative's wooden warehouses and replaced them with grey concrete collective warehouses. These massive rectangular buildings now stood vandalised and destroyed, grasses growing from their floors.

Along the shoreline lay old wooden skiffs and fishing boats, long abandoned. Some lay partly submerged in the shallow waters offshore or alongside the concrete wharfs. Reeds grew in abundance and behind the weeds more grasses and wildflowers in which orb spiders had spun countless perfect webs which glistened in the angular morning light. From Kihelkonna I could hear the faint sound of ringing church bells. I investigated the abandoned boats, looking for a souvenir, and tried to remove the old wooden wheel from one of them but my Roadtrek's tool kit wasn't complete enough to get through the accumulated years of rust.

The drive back to Kihelkonna was even more enchanting because now I was driving towards the sun and the cobbles shone and sparkled as if covered in quartz dust. At the end of the road stood the 60 metre high steeple of Kihelkonna church, set apart from the town itself. I parked nearby and as I approached, two starlings in the eaves of the church erupted into a turbulent

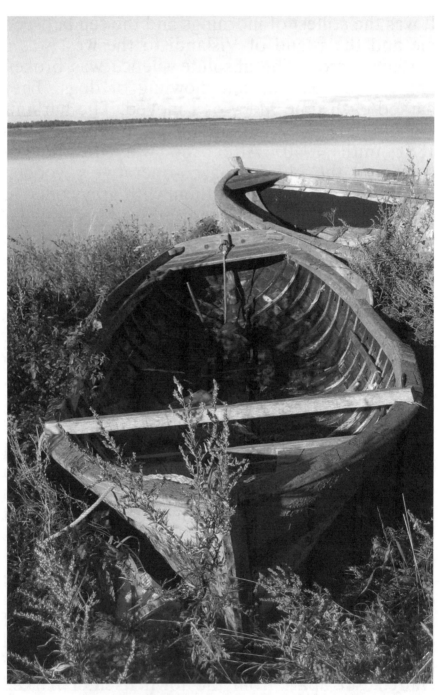

ALONG THE SHORELINE LAY OLD WOODEN SKIFFS
AND FISHING BOATS, LONG ABANDONED

bickering aerial combat, and fell like lead weights towards the lush grass below, then broke apart and flew off just before what had looked like an inevitable collision with the ground. The current belfry was built only a little over 100 years ago and doubled as a lighthouse. The church's old bell tower is still where it always was 100 metres away in a field. The separation of church and bell tower was once common here.

Much vernacular architecture survives in Kihelkonna as do more recent grey-brick monstrosities. Abandoned by one grey-brick square building was a rusting green Polski Fiat. A Japanese installation artist could not have conjured up a better combination. And even here, at 9 a.m. on a Sunday morning there were intoxicated men, young and old, with vodka bottles, marring the peace and serenity.

*   *   *

I'd seen signs further back on Saaremaa to a German cemetery. As cotton-wool, cumulus clouds appeared overhead I took a series of dirt roads south through woodland following the signs towards the Sõrve peninsula.

In 1939 Germany and Russia signed the secret Molotov-Ribbentrop pact in which Germany 'gave' Finland and the Baltic states, beginning with Estonia, to Russia. In 1939 Russia invaded Finland but withdrew from most of it a few months later. In 1940 they occupied Estonia more successfully and the country was incorporated into the Soviet Union. In 1941 Hitler reneged on his infamous treaty with Stalin and Germany occupied Estonia,

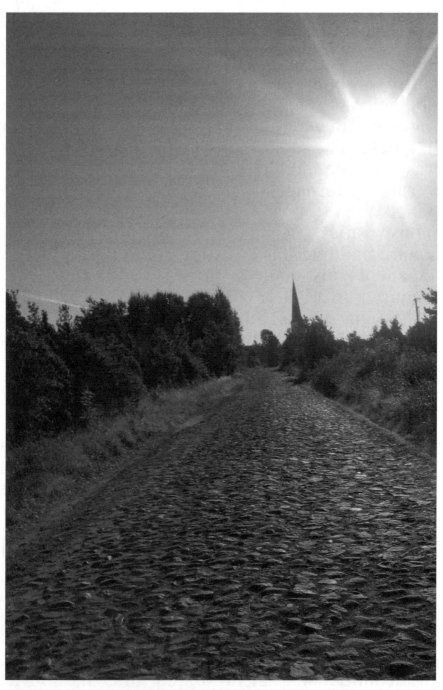

THE COBBLES SHONE AND SPARKLED AS IF COVERED
IN QUARTZ DUST

including Saaremaa.

They stayed until, the sign at Tehumardi told me, the 8th of November 1944 when the Red Army breached this last German stronghold in Estonia and defeated their enemy.

Near the battle site is an angular, brutal, monolith, a cement and dolomite memorial to that battle. Impassive, determined, square-jawed faces look immutably towards the sea and in the morning light it was more moving, more thought-provoking than any other man-made structure I saw on the island.

In the aftermath, virtually all of Saaremaa's and the mainland's residents of Swedish ancestry fled to Sweden. In Stockholm Ake had told me that many of these refugees became cattle artificial inseminators.

The Soviets placed severe restrictions on movement on Saaremaa and especially on the Sõrve peninsula which became an exclusion zone and a major Soviet submarine base. Deportations decimated the local population and those who remained needed permits to visit the peninsula. As I strolled round, lost in thought about the Soviet rule, and the anger of the man at the ferry terminal, still so keenly felt, berries were ripening on the juniper bushes and the sandy beach looked innocent. I wandered south and at a rocky section, lifted rocks and tried in vain to catch crayfish. Further down the beach Macy was preoccupied by her own discovery—a decomposing grey seal, perhaps three days dead.

In the main town of Kuressaare, known until 1917 as Arensburg, there's a picture postcard sand-coloured medieval stone castle with a deep

145

moat, surrounded by old housing stock—Empire and Art Nouveau villas and cobbled streets—all with grey-brick buildings interspersed. It's gearing up for increased tourism. The 'John Bull Pub' now occupies a traditional wooden house next to the castle and terraced restaurants circle the parking area.

We walked the star-shaped system of earthworks that girdle the castle's deep moat and Macy survived an encounter with a tough black tom-cat with white spats, whose territory she had entered. Throughout Estonia, on the mainland and here on Saaremaa, wherever we walked there were countless feral cats.

There was what turned out to be a five-hour queue for the ferry back to the mainland. Each arriving ferry disgorged exactly 12 tour buses, almost all from Latvia, and I seldom moved any further forward because other cars skipped the line and boarded the boats. I never learned whether this was through bribery or buying tickets with guaranteed return times.

Others were delayed as long as I was and I talked cars with a tattooed guy with a number one haircut, and trees with a more academic man— round face, round glasses, round belly, an all-rounder. Both spoke excellent English compared to my single-word Estonian vocabulary, 'Tere,' hello.

The academic man was not, in fact, an academic. He worked for the Estonian State Bank in Tallinn and I asked him with whom amongst the Baltic people he identified most.

'We are hard-working people, perhaps a little boring but we are rational, careful. It was difficult when we banned the rouble and replaced it with the kroon but it worked. We were sensible when we employed a Swedish banker. He was only the deputy but those of us at the bank knew he made decisions for us.'

At Ismo's Ruunawere Hotell near Tallinn there's a black granite tombstone on the front lawn. When I asked him what it said on the marker, he explained, 'The Old Rouble—Born 1940—Died 1992.' Ismo had told me a little about the Estonian economy so I knew what the banker in the ferry queue was referring to.

'Are you saying you identify with the Swedes?' I asked.

'I think we are a Scandinavian people,' he answered and I asked about corruption. Surely in the chaos of change from a command to a market economy, corruption thrived here as it did elsewhere in the former Soviet Union.

'You see the trees on Muhu and Saaremaa? Did you see how much young the forest is? The young forests were once farms. The Soviets destroyed farming and that is most difficult to repair. That is the lasting legacy of the Soviet era. Yes, there is corruption.'

He continued, 'After the Soviet times land was returned to the children of historical owners. In Soviet times the forests were owned by the State but now they are owned by absent people who don't care about the land and are interested in money. They cut the trees and sell them. Its called 'black' timber. They plant nothing and the government does nothing because it cannot check what is happening. Much of the logging in Estonia is illegal. You ask about corruption. The tree

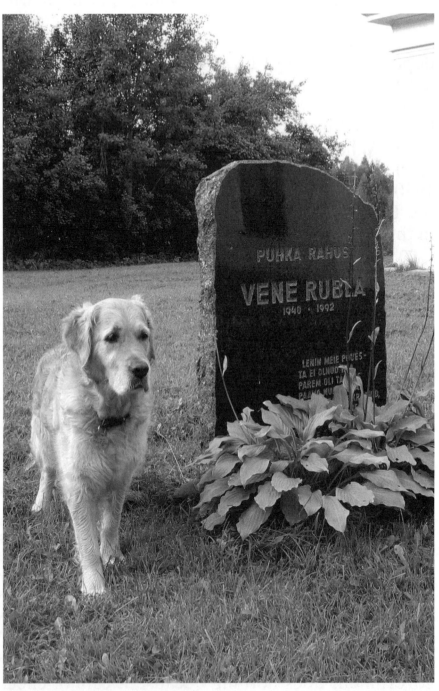

THE GRAVE OF THE OLD ROUBLE—BORN 1940—
DIED 1992

cutting is illegal but who is buying the trees? Who is being corrupt? Sweden and Finland.'

I asked about the EU and he paused, then with an almost embarrassed half-smile he lowered his head and looked at me.

'I am a banker. My mind tells me what is good for my country. My history tells me another story. It is impossible for you to understand. We were raped by one power. Now another has seduced us. But they both are after the same thing, what we can do for them not what they can do for us. Is it difficult to understand we just want to be us?'

*　　　*　　　*

After returning from Saaremaa to the mainland Macy and I spent the afternoon in and around the attractive old town of Haapsalu. It wasn't far from the ferry port which linked Estonia to the Baltic island of Hiiumaa. There were Falck guards there too, patrolling in vehicles marked with their logo, 'Falck Off!' OK, I lie, but Falck guards were ubiquitous.

Leaving Tallinn the day before, I saw a Falck-uniformed patrol at a school crossing. 'Falck Safely' said the school-crossing sign. Or was it 'Falck With Us'? 'Falck This Way'? 'Don't Falck With Us'? Outside town I saw my first ever stork in a nest, atop a purpose-built tripod tower. In the park by Haapsalu's Africa Beach, Macy play-bowed and made instant friends with a wire-haired dachshund-like little dog and they raced figure eights on the grass and on the sand. This was the first dog she had met in Estonia that hadn't tried to kill her.

149

Haapsalu is an agreeable place, a marketable town waiting to be transformed. It has a ruined Gothic castle and a warehouse of a cathedral but more important, there are rows of low painted wooden houses radiating from the circular market square. Some time in the near future Haapsalu will draw the tourists from Tallinn as Porvoo draws them from Helsinki.

*　　　　*　　　　*

When I returned to Ruunawere Hotell that evening the guests were helping Ismo stack firewood that had arrived during the day. Fact: it takes seven drunk Finns, one sober visitor and one hotelier less than three hours to move and neatly stack 10,000, 30-centimetre-long split birch logs. My reward was a one per cent commission: 100 of those perfect white-barked gems which are now stacked at home beside my fireplace, sacrificed ever so occasionally.

*　　　　*　　　　*

The Tallinn Zoo sits in the western suburbs of the Estonian capital and was founded in 1937 to accommodate a baby lynx the Estonian Rifleman's Society didn't know what to do with after they had won it at a shooting championship in Helsinki. I now have several ties in different colours with that lynx on it, gifts from the museum director, Mati Kaal.

In Sweden I'd received a telephone call from my dentist, Peter Kertész. Knowing I was going to be in Tallinn, he asked if I'd visit the zoo and measure

150

the width of a tusk he had removed from an elephant when he had been in Tallinn two days previously. The zoo still had the bits of tusk. Peter does people Mondays to Thursdays and non-people on Fridays. He'd emailed Mati and arranged my visit.

Mati met me at the gate with his librarian, Tiiu, who would be our translator for the day. They caught me just as I had found yet another tick—dead—on Macy and removed it. Mati's English was good and his German excellent. During the Soviet era, when contact with western zoos was forbidden, he had frequent meetings and exchanges with East German curators.

When the Iron Curtain was lifted and he was able to visit the West he discovered that his fluent German was not as useful as he thought it would be. In Copenhagen, the local curator understood German but asked Mati to speak only in English. Tiiu's English was more than just excellent. She's translated Jerome's *Three Men in a Boat*—and other books—into Estonian.

'The parking lot is not guarded. Your wonderful vehicle will be safer inside the gate,' Tiiu explained. She told me they had all my books in the zoo library. I was seriously impressed as I had no idea so many were even translated into Estonian.

I don't like zoos. I feel uncomfortable seeing animals in small enclosures but this visit turned out to be a learning experience. I was introduced to a 38-year-old black rhinoceros, who's been terrified of female rhinoceroses ever since one accidentally crushed his willy 19 years ago. I met the zoo vet who had just completed a post-mortem

151

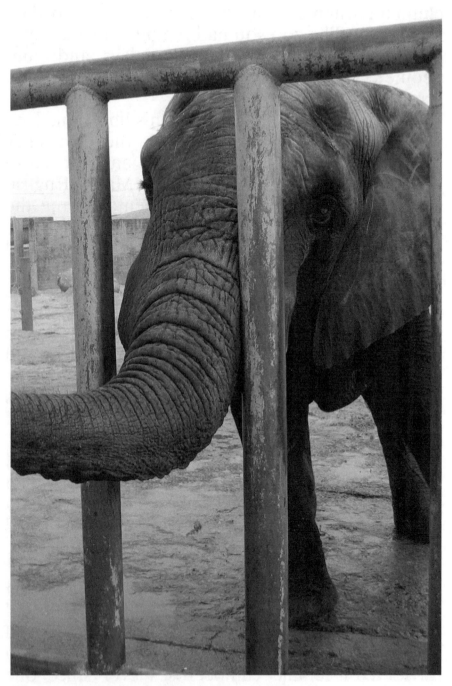

CARL THE ESTONIAN BULL ELEPHANT

on an elk which died from eating plastic, the most common cause of death at the zoo.

Peter Kertész tells me he knows of three Nile hippopotami in European zoos that died from swallowing tennis balls. For some reason visitors think that the hippos would like the balls to play with. As we walked past the long-tailed goral from the Amur region of Siberia, an animal in a classification between mountain goat and antelope, Mati explained that their numbers surprisingly had declined even though their predators, Siberian tigers, were slowly becoming extinct. Grey wolves entered the empty niche previously occupied by the tigers and were ravaging the goral population.

The zoo's young, athletic, education director was recovering from a serious attack by a large guarding dog, a Caucasian Owtcharka, which had mauled his face. I was grateful for the opportunity to meet him because I could tell him how much I liked the pictographs he'd designed for the animal enclosure labels. A quick read is enough to learn about the social life of an animal, its natural habitat, what time of the day it's active, what it eats, its life span, when it mates, the length of gestation and the size of an average litter. Other pictographs explain length, height and weight, whether it's under 'protection', 'endangered' or on the 'red list' of world conservation. Good stuff.

I'd promised Peter I'd get measurements on the tusk, the second one he'd extracted from Carl, a massive bull elephant. Tusks easily get damaged in zoos because of the environment the elephants live in. Tusks are actually continually growing incisor teeth deeply embedded in the maxilla bone and

153

their ivory is nothing more than dentine. The pulp in the central canal produces and lays down new dentine, enabling the tusk to grow. When operating on elephant tusks Peter occasionally finds large pearls of dentine in the pulp. When he does he knows there has been a previous episode of inflammation and this dentine pearl was formed in response to that.

If the pulp cavity is not exposed it may only need smoothing with a very large tungsten burr. If there's more serious damage, but it's been done relatively recently and there's no infection, the tusk can be saved by carrying out a form of pulp treatment to keep the pulp alive and healthy by encouraging the formation of an ivory bridge to wall off the remaining healthy pulp. This is done by cutting and cleaning the pulp back a considerable distance then plugging the canal by cementing a resin rod into it. There's a good success rate in young elephants but a miserable one in older bulls. Their naturally aggressive behaviour leads to inevitable further tusk damage. If deep infection develops in the pulp cavity or the maxillary bone itself, the tusk needs extraction.

Infection is every bit as painful to an elephant as an infected tooth is to us. Antibiotics give short-term relief but extraction is the only way to resolve chronic infection. Peter has carried out more pulp treatments and tusk extractions on more elephants than any other person, dentist or veterinarian.

Using instruments Peter had made for the purpose, he reamed out Carl's pulp canal with giant drills until the tusk wall was thin enough to section into parallel strips, then he removed a strip at a time using special splitters, elevators and forceps. Each parallel strip I examined was around 10 centimetres wide and 70 centimetres long. Carl was contentedly munching his grass when I saw him, pain-free.

We walked through the goat hills and paddocks, the most complete in the world outside San Diego Zoo, and finally reached the place I really wanted to see, the mink enclosure. Here was a striking reason for a modern zoo. Before we in the West even realised how serious the problem was, Mati and his colleagues were trying to save the European mink from imminent extinction.

The European mink looks almost identical to the American mink but they are very distant relatives, so genetically dissimilar that their matings are sterile. The European mink is, in fact close kin to European and Siberian polecats. Matings with either of those species result in live litters. The fact that it looks so like the American mink is simply a brilliant example of adaptive convergence, that way in which two different species end up looking and behaving remarkably similarly because they both inhabit the same ecological niche. In this instance it's a semi-aquatic lifestyle amongst the deep vegetation of river banks and lakesides eating fish, molluscs, frogs, small mammals, crayfish and insects.

A century ago the European mink thrived across the continent but in the twentieth century their numbers dwindled, first slowly, then worryingly fast. The last wild individuals in Lithuania were seen in 1979, in Finland in 1992, in Latvia in 1993. They probably became extinct in Estonia three years later. During the twentieth century the species became extinct in 20 European countries.

Today there's a small remnant population on the Spanish-French border, another—perhaps—on the Romania-Moldova border and a larger one in north-west Russia, where it is still legal to hunt them. Mati's mink come from the Russian enclave.

I asked what was driving the European mink to extinction and he replied that there was now such a crisis it was too late to discover exactly what it was. Certainly habitat loss was one reason. In the former Soviet Union there was water pollution and heavy metals, PCBs and organophosphates all affect breeding rates. A parvovirus called ADV—a viral relative of viral enteritis in cats and canine parvovirus in dogs—wiped out many of them. So did road traffic when numbers were still large, but it's the American mink, an exotic, aggressive invader who's perhaps the major cause of the annihilation of European mink. To paraphrase what Mati told me, American mink were screwing the European mink to extinction.

Mink are small animals. Females weigh around half a kilo while males grow up to twice that size. American mink, originally brought to Europe in 1926 for fur farming, are more adaptive and creative than European mink, and quickly colonise any environment with potential. European mink on the other hand are rigid in their ways, set in their habits. When my son Ben spent a year on the remote Scottish island of Taransay, a mile into the rough northern Atlantic off the island of Lewes and Harris, in the Western Isles of Scotland, I was amazed when I visited him to learn that his dog Inca amused herself by chasing feral mink. These were fur farm American mink that escaped, swam through the strong currents to Taransay and

156

survived by predating bird eggs. On that one island alone there are thousands.

The American's trump card is its sexual precocity. American females come into their receptive spring oestrus sooner. That activates the males who mate with them, and as soon as the Europeans come into oestrus they screw them too before the male Europeans have a chance. The American females give birth to viable litters but the European females' half-American foetuses stop growing, die and their tissue is 'resorbed' or broken down and eliminated. By then it's too late for the European males. Oestrus is over.

The consequence is instantaneous zero growth in the European mink population. As their life expectancy in the wild is around six years, it takes the shortest of time for the species to reach the edge of extinction or drop over it.

At Tallinn Mati has set up a rehab centre where zoo-bred European mink are being trained to forage and fend for themselves. The island of Hiiumaa off the coast of Haavsalu was cleared of American mink, and European mink bred and trained at the Tallinn Zoo have been released there. If this is successful, the same will be attempted on the island of Saaremaa. Mati's colleague Tiit Maran calculated that to preserve genetic diversity they need 400 to 500 individuals but the decimation of the species was so rapid there was no time to collect that many, let alone find zoos willing to participate in their Noah's Ark scheme. There was no money either. When the Soviet Union collapsed the zoo's funds dried up.

In 1991, eight of the Tallinn mink died from digestive disorders probably caused by poor food quality. Finances didn't improve until the Helsinki and Ahtari Zoos in Finland injected needed funds. Mati has around 100 breeding European mink at the zoo now, and there are another 100 spread around 15 other zoos. That's it. The entire world population of captive European mink. If the Hiiumaa project fails, the species has little chance of natural survival.

*   *   *

In 1793, in the early years of the French Revolution, France's National Convention abolished the old calendar. Henceforth each year would begin at midnight on the autumn equinox. Midnight, 22 September 1792 was the beginning of Year One. New weeks had 10 days and there were three weeks to each of the 12 new months: Vendemaire (harvest), Brumaire (mist), Frimaire (frost), Nivose (snow), Pluviose (rain), Ventose (wind), Germinal (seeds), Floreal (flowers), Prairial (haymaking), Messidor (reaping), Thermidor (heat) and Fructidor (fruits). Such is the pompous idiocy of revolution.

The Republican calendar lasted 14 years but 200 years later revolutionaries continued to enact the absurd. I was reminded of this French folly when I commented to Mati that it was odd to see a European jay in his bird collection. Jays nest within 50 metres of my veterinary clinic in London.

'The jay was officially prohibited from the zoo in Soviet times,' he told me. When I asked why, he told me that it was decided that the four centimetre-square patch of blue on their wings might become a focus for Estonian nationalism.

The aesthetically beautiful state flag is white, black and blue.

When the writer Adam Nicolson travelled through Tallinn in 1984, in the twilight years of the Soviet Empire, he said that Tallinn 'reeks of bourgeois cosiness . . . no wonder over a million Russians come to Tallinn as tourists each year. It acts as a surrogate West.' Then he noticed there was something fake about it. Simply hoisting the white, blue and black flag, he discovered, condemned you to five years' imprisonment and forced labour.

Thinking of all the square grey-brick homes I'd seen on my drive through Estonia, I asked why the new buildings in the countryside weren't built in traditional styles and Mati explained that the Soviets did not permit vernacular architecture. It might become a focus for nationalism. He told me that after the Moscow Olympics in 1980 what little money there had been for the zoo dried up. To pay for the Olympics, Moscow placed a ten-year ban on building or renewing any 'cultural facilities' and that included improvements to his zoo.

'During the Soviet era an army of Party bureaucrats monopolised life. They glorified their own aesthetics and tried to control children from birth through nurseries and youth movements. They censored what could be heard but we listened to Helsinki. They had contempt for individuals. Any means justified their goal. Those Estonians who left the country moved away to escape the system, not because of poverty. They kept their nationalism alive in your country and now their children are returning. It will take three generations to recover from the Soviet Union,'

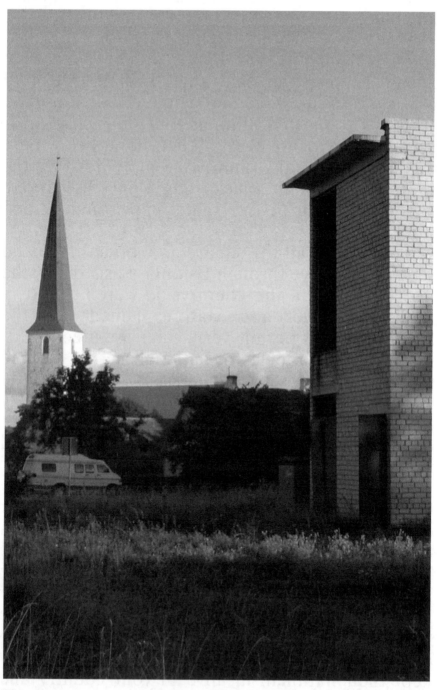

THE OLD AND THE NEW ARCHITECTURE OF
ESTONIA

Mati explained through Tiiu.

'What about the EU?' I asked.

Mati replied that the choice was between 'bad' and 'very bad'.

Tiiu added, 'We've had enough experience with Unions. The Soviet Union and now the European Union. Our natural inclination was not to become part of another Union. Sharing Europe's values means we must now share the European Union's high prices. We would prefer to be Estonia but we are only small and that is impossible.'

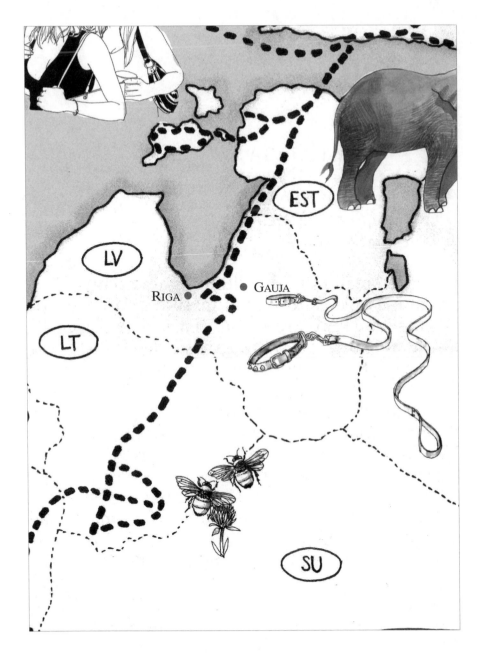

CHAPTER FIVE

LATVIA

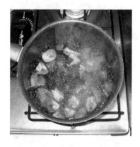

LATVIA

People per square kilometre	*35*
Dogs per square kilometre	*4*
Two-headed dogs	*1*

Latvia is small but her wildlife is abundant. There are more wolves here than in all of 'Old Europe' combined. There are just as many lynx—over 400 of them—but I was here to visit the Baltic's only true city, Riga, and to encounter a two-headed dog.

It had rained heavily overnight. I'd stopped in Parnu, Estonia's seaside resort town, but wherever I walked Owtcharkas threw themselves at fences, barking and growling obscenities, desperate to eviscerate my dog as she ambled past, so I continued south leaving the empty E67 main road, taking the virtually unused old coastal road past sleepy agricultural settlements and waterside villas.

The beautiful Baltic beaches were as empty as the roads. I'd stopped for a walk at Kabli Nature Trail and shortly after I arrived, a convoy of three other cars, all 4WDs, stopped too and their occupants joined the trail. Hearing me speaking English to Macy, one of them, a full-figured woman with blue eyes and black hair came over.

'Hello. What are you doing so far away from a major city?' she asked, with obvious curiosity. I explained that I was mostly avoiding cities and travelling through the countryside.

'What is your speciality?' she asked. It seemed to her that only an 'ologist' would do what I was doing. She was a hydrologist, returning to Parnu from a scientific meeting in Riga.

*   *   *

At Krapi, just north of the Latvian border I camped on State Forest Management land, where firewood was free and fresh water on tap. The evening had cooled and there were no mosquitoes. Sitting alone in mature pine woods, smelling the scent of autumn, gazing at a roaring birch fire and listening to the waves breaking on the shore reminded me of camping on the shores of Lake Michigan. There, Macy had taken off after forest life and been lost in the woods for two agonising hours, but here she was content to lie by my side and fire gaze with me.

Overnight, another camper, from Finland in a vast Hymer motorhome, had joined me and parked at the opposite end of the campsite. He'd laid a place for his accompanying cat at the outdoor table he'd set up for breakfast—separate food and milk bowls—and provided her with her own cardboard container to sit on so she wouldn't get damp when she jumped down to the rain-sodden ground. I offered a good morning 'Hei' but couldn't make eye contact with him.

The flat expansive beach at Krapi was superb, stretching as far as the eye could see in both directions. The end nearest the woods was covered in hillocks of marram grass standing like dark green gumdrops on a sea of golden sand. In the sharp, early morning sunlight the Baltic was a cold midnight blue. Macy found driftwood to retrieve and waded in the rolling surf, in pools and in freshwater rivulets carrying last night's rainfall from the surrounding forest into the sea.

*   *   *

At the Latvian border crossing I was given a straight-backed full salute by a stern fluorescent-red-haired female border guard who carefully inspected my vehicle's documents. Her Latvian sounded like Russian to my ears. My Latvian is as extensive as my Estonian—'*Labdien*' or 'hello'. The E67, a vast, unending construction site now called the Via Baltica hugs the coast until just north of Riga.

Unlike in Estonia, where straw was baled, here it was piled in traditional old haystacks. Laika-like dogs wandered the highway's edge playing dodgem with the road traffic and the broadcaster on the only radio station I could find sounded so morose, so depressed that I turned him off and hid the kitchen knives in case Macy had been listening.

As in Estonia, buildings were built with grey bricks although there were now occasional buildings of red brick too. The women I saw were Ohio-fat. The landscape was a mosaic of forest, occasional farmland and abandoned meadows reverting to bush and woodland. Close to 20 years after the end of the Soviet era and it was obvious that the governments here and in Estonia don't yet have a policy for these abandoned lands. At least the cows looked striking, like shiny bovine Irish setters. Their heads and legs are darker and they are officially called Latvian Browns. These good-lookers make up almost three-quarters of the cows in Latvia.

*   *   *

Riga is big, brash, flashy, cosmopolitan, sophisticated—certainly not dourly Baltic. It bustled. I parked near the National Theatre and took Macy for a walk through the adjacent park and then past the Emporio Armani on Elizabeth Street, past the TGI Friday restaurant in the Old Town, through Cathedral Square and Castle Square to Town Hall Square where the gilded, ornamented, fourteenth-century neoclassical Town Hall, reconstructed from scratch in the 1990s, squats like an overdressed red wedding cake. I returned Macy to the Roadtrek and headed off to the Paul Stradins Museum of the History of Medicine, my real reason for visiting Riga. This is where I would see the two-headed dog.

You enter the museum through a cellar where, for one lat (somewhat less than a euro) a creepy woman sells you a ticket then forbids you to enter until she takes back the ticket and stamps it. Another creepy old woman standing two metres away blocks your entry until she inspects the green stamp she watched the first creepy woman stamp. Clones of these crones sat impassively in every room in the museum. I was the only visitor.

I wasn't interested in the basement dioramas of cavemen trepanning skulls or, on the next floor,

167

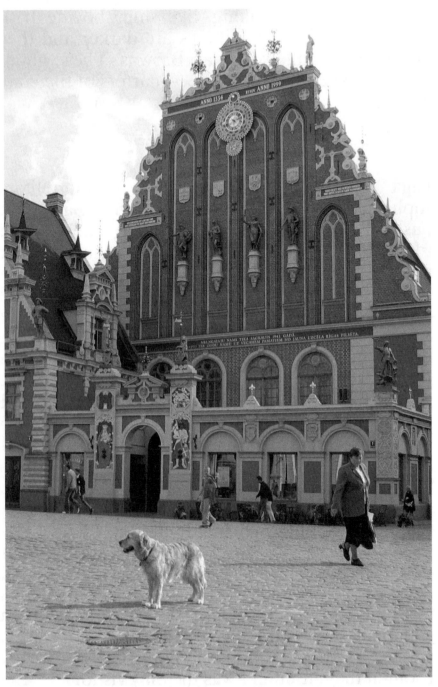

THE BEAUTIFUL RECONSTRUCTED TOWN HALL IN
RIGA

medieval medical instruments, although seeing Pasteur's, Koch's, Metchnikoff's and Roentgen's scientific equipment on higher floors of the house was actually quite interesting. I made my way to the top floor, 'Soviet Medicine' and there it was, in the middle of the room in a raised rectangular glass case: the two-headed dog.

Lying sphinx-like on a black marble base was a fawn-coloured, erect-eared, German shepherd-like dog of around 25 kilograms. Straddling its shoulders were the forequarters of another, smaller dog. That little dog had erect ears too, and a mostly black face with a white neck, chest and legs. When it was once whole, before it was cut in two and its head was surgically grafted on to the larger dog it probably weighed 6 or 7 kilograms. The two-headed dog was the consequence of live animal experimental surgery carried out in the early 1950s at Moscow State University by Vladimir Petrovich Demikhov.

Examining the taxidermist's work, I was appalled to think how these dogs suffered. The small dog's body had been amputated behind its shoulders, a large hole had been made in the bigger dog's back and their blood vessels and then muscles and skin grafted together. Demikhov wanted to see whether the larger dog's internal organs could sustain life in the smaller dog, whether the small dog's brain could be kept alive. An apocryphal story tells that upon awakening from anaesthesia the large dog was so disturbed to find another dog straddling its neck that it circled like a dervish trying to bite it. If you believe the story, then Demikhov's vascular surgery was so successful the smaller dog got equally enraged and

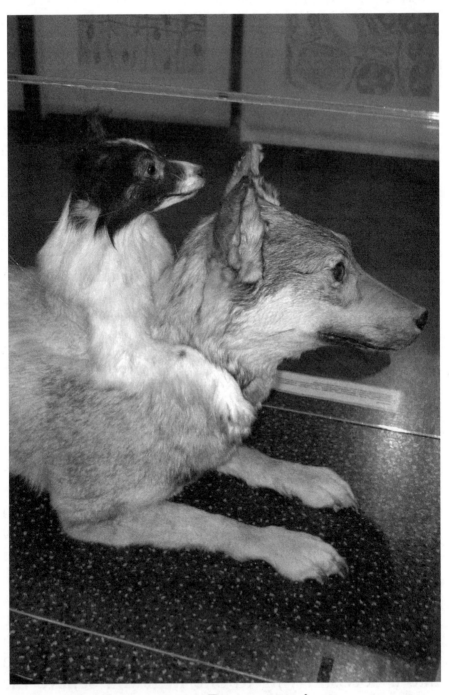

VLADIMIR PETROVICH DEMIKHOV'S TWO-HEADED
DOG

bit back.

I borrowed a copy of *Experimental Transplantation of Vital Organs*, Demikhov's text published in English translation in 1962, from the library, but there was no specific mention of this two-headed dog. He sacrificed hundreds of other dogs in his experimental organ transplantations.

The Wellcome Institute for the History of Medicine in London holds Witness Seminars in which it gathers witnesses to significant medical events to tell their stories. Ten years ago it held a Witness Seminar on early heart transplant surgery in the UK. Professor Donald Longmore recounted doing heart-lung transplants in 1963 at the Royal Veterinary College in London, dog to sheep, sheep to dog, sheep to pig. Dr Alan Gilston, who was Senior Consultant Anaesthesiologist at the National Heart Hospital, reminded him that the first transplant was a pig heart transplant at his hospital. 'I remember chasing piggy round the corridors of the hospital. I had never anaesthetised a pig before, but that wasn't terribly successful, so we didn't have the press in on that.'

I don't see humour, as I suspect Gilston did, in 'chasing piggy round the corridors'. I see the fear the pig endured as it tried to evade capture. I don't see the advancement of science in Demikhov's two-headed dog. I see inhumane suffering. But both of these men advanced science. They developed new surgical techniques we now consider routine. Lives have been saved—human and animal lives including other dogs because of what they did.

In 1968, when dog-to-dog heart transplants were being carried out under Home Office licence at

171

the Royal Veterinary College I too was doing transplant surgery. At the Ontario Veterinary College, my professor of surgery Jim Archibald employed his favourite students during the summer break. I was one of them and he had us perfecting our vascular surgery skills by taking a kidney from a dog's belly and transplanting it into the dog's neck, between the jugular vein and the carotid artery.

I worked with a team operating for eight hours at a time on pregnant sows. We opened their abdomens, opened their wombs, opened the piglet's chests and made holes in their diaphragms then sewed them all up. Days later the sows gave birth, in the presence of obstetricians, to piglets with holes in their diaphragms. At that time, human babies born with congenital holes in their diaphragms invariably died. The obstetrical team tried to devise methods to keep the piglets alive long enough for paediatric surgeons to intervene and operate.

The value for me in doing these experiments was that I became a better surgeon faster and learned from operating on these animals rather than on people's pets. I wouldn't do these things today, not because I disagree with them. I have no problem with acute, non-survival experiments carried out on animals under full anaesthesia, animals that before surgery have been housed and cared for in conditions that are appropriate for their emotional and physical well-being.

No, I wouldn't because after working so intimately with animals for so long I know them too well. I wince when a pup yips when I insert an identifying microchip! Like most other vets my

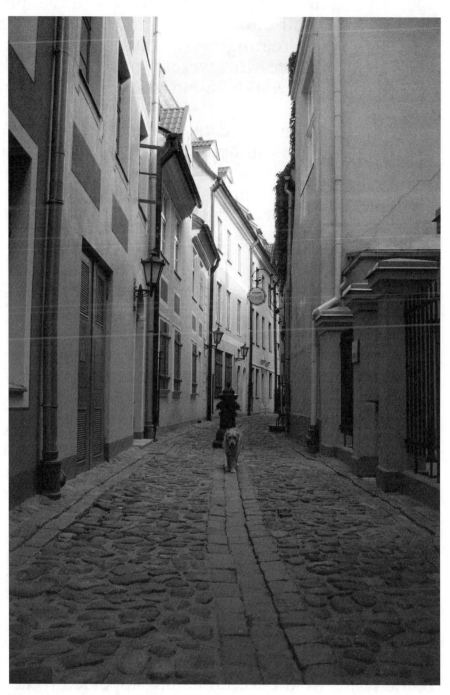

THE NARROW COBBLED BACKSTREETS OF OLD RIGA

age, I've gone soft. Demikhov was a callous bastard. He had no feelings for the dogs he operated on. Creating a two-headed dog was hubris, not science. But were it not for bastards like him there would be no transplant surgery today.

While I contemplated these pathetic dogs, the room's guardian got up and went to a hallway cupboard where she had a tea kettle. I took that opportunity to take photos of the exhibit, scamper down the stone stairs and depart.

*   *   *

There's a terrific open-air ethnographic museum just a few kilometres outside Riga, on the road to Sigulda and the Gauja National Park where I planned to stay that evening. Its grounds are expansive and wooded, much like Stockholm's Skansen. As at Skansen, the displays make nineteenth-century rural life seem charming and idyllic. The kitchen gardens were filled with medicinal herbs, the apple trees were bounteous with red fruit and the naive paintings on the church ceilings exuded a simple, innocent charm. I thought it odd however that although Jews were the second largest ethnic group in nineteenth-century Latvia there was no historical evidence of them here.

Macy thought the new four-lane highway heading north-east from Riga was an absolute pleasure. The corrugated surfaces of the other Baltic roads we'd covered hadn't appealed to her. The surrounding pine forest all the way to Sigulda was majestic and it took no time to arrive there and find a campsite beside the Gaujas River. The weather remained sunny and fresh, perfect for walking and we investigated the river banks where the sand was littered with rabbit footprints and large freshwater clam shells. Then we took to the park's nature trails.

The Gauja National Park website baldly states, 'Maintain the serenity of nature and don't disturb other visitors. Leave your dog(s) in your car.' They are unaware that western European dogs, unlike their Eastern European counterparts, don't perpetually bark, growl and threaten imminent death to whoever they see. Macy went with me. Not a single person complained. Then again, during the next two hours we didn't meet a single person.

The following morning we climbed the hundreds of wooden steps on a nature trail that wends its way up from the river to Sigulda and wandered through town. It was 8 a.m. and in the misty Baltic light, surrounded by the scent of ripe apples, yellow birch leaves fell languidly, like slowly descending butterflies. I counted 34 women with witches' brooms sweeping leaves on the streets. Drunks were already lurching down the roads. I visited the local Elvi supermarket and stocked up on bread and cheese. Shoppers looked phlegmatic, passive, insular, sad.

Back on the E67 I was sad too, heading inland towards the border with Lithuania. There's something soothing about the seashore. Julia, who was born by the sea finds no special comfort in it. Macy and I thrive on it. At a long-distance lorry park, men were giving their giant canine companions—protection dogs—morning walks.

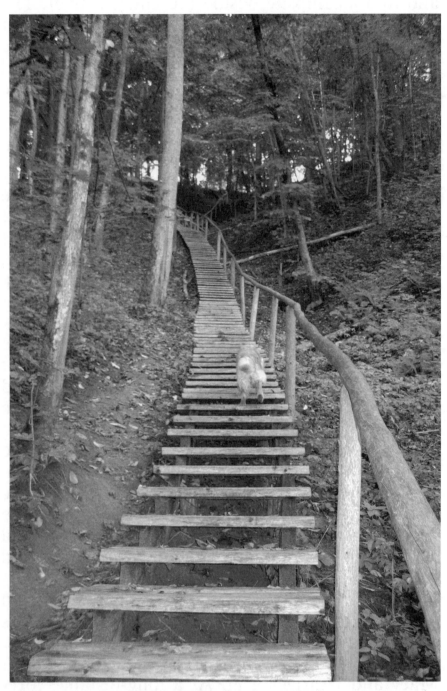

THE HUNDREDS OF WOODEN STEPS ON A NATURE TRAIL

People with empty, small plastic buckets walked along the roadside and I assumed they were either berry or mushroom pickers. The land was flat and this highway too was a constantly unfolding construction site.

I didn't get a feel for Latvia. My visit was shorter than I would have wanted but I had an appointment to keep in Kaunas, Lithuania. I don't know if there is such a thing as a Latvian national character. The ethnographic museum portrays a rural culture but over a third of the country's entire population lives in Riga alone and what is that city's culture? Riga was built by the Germans and Poles, occupied by the Swedes and Lithuanians and made wealthy by its Jewish merchants. Ethnic Russians make up half of its citizens. It's easy to forget that its miles of Art Nouveau architecture stand as a tribute to its wealth during the Russian Empire. It was, after all, Russia's biggest port. It's easy to forget too, that it was, in its essence, a Jewish mercantile city. Monuments to that heritage were destroyed by the Germans, disregarded by the Soviets and now seem to be forgotten by the Latvians. I left not knowing what to think.

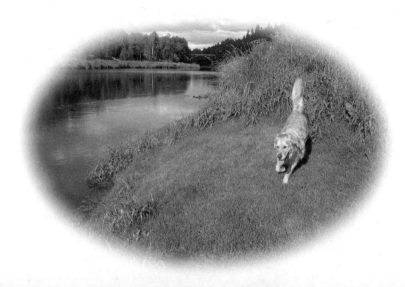

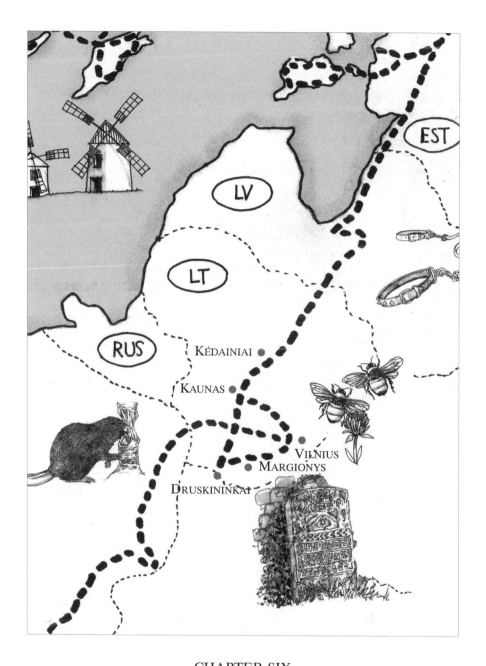

CHAPTER SIX

LITHUANIA

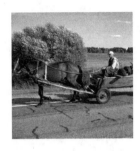

LITHUANIA

People per square kilometre	*53*
Dogs per square kilometre	*6*
Jews per square kilometre	*One twentieth of one*

'Lithuania, there is no money. Lithuanians don't know how to work. They only concerned with your money. There is old Lithuanian saying: "Every Lithuanian hopes his neighbour's horse dies."' Andreas, who cleans houses in London, told me before I left on this trip.

If that were to happen there would be a lot of surplus horse meat in Lithuania. As soon as I crossed the border from Latvia they were everywhere, pulling carts on the roads, pulling ploughs in the fields, unhitched from carts while parties of people filled sacks with potatoes or just standing stoically in green fields, tethered or hobbled, waiting to be called upon for more work.

As elsewhere the border guards were fascinated by my Roadtrek but here the three young uniformed men were enamoured with Macy too.

'Name?' The square-faced, square-jawed, square-eyed guard asked.

'Fogle,' I answered.

'No. Name. Retriever.'

'Macy,' I said and he hand signalled to ask

whether he could give her something.

'Maaaaacy,' he cooed, as if he'd met the woman of his dreams. It was a pleasant welcome to Lithuania.

I didn't know exactly what to expect, or for that matter how I'd feel visiting this country. I knew it had been the home of my ancestors for at least 300 years, probably longer. My maternal great-great-great-great-great-great-grandfather was born in Vilnius in 1690. In my mother's family there is a photo of his great-great-grandson, Reuven Breslin, born in 1801, two years after Napoleon Bonaparte entered Paris and ended the French Revolution.

It was Reuven's generation who were the first to be given new modern surnames. Much more recently, my father's mother, Leah Bernard, was born somewhere in these lands in 1876 and lived here long enough to remember going on rent collecting rounds with her inn keeper father. All of my parents' families, the Fogles, Bernards, Breslins and Papernicks had left this region of Europe two generations before the Germans arrived in 1941. My extended families were not directly affected by their murderous occupation.

*   *   *

I was in the heartland of the Great European Plain. The black soil looked wonderfully fertile and, on this sunny day with full hay-ricks in the fields, milk-churns by the roadside, horse-drawn carts on the highway and tethered cows and hobbled horses in the meadows, it was as if I had stepped back into a lost and idyllic world. Most fields had one or two cows but some had herds, all of them chained out on tethers. As in Estonia and Latvia, there were no restricting fences along the roads for financial rather than aesthetic reasons.

Occasionally I'd see a decrepit tractor, looking as though it had emerged from the film set of *The Grapes of Wrath*, belching black diesel fumes as the driver ploughed a field. More often fields were being worked by a man with a hand-held plough pulled by a single sturdy, well-kept Baltic pony. I stopped at one field to watch a woman sitting on a three-legged wooden stool milking a tethered black cow, squirting the warm liquid straight into a small churn. When she finished she moved on to her other cow, a brown one, and milked it into another small aluminium churn. All the while her husband drove up and down the end of the field on a rickety rust-coloured tractor.

In some fields the straw had been hand-raked into small piles the size of coffins. In one of these fields a horse-drawn cart was being walked to each pile and I watched the farmer fork the straw on to the flat cart. In another I watched two men building the last of three haystacks, an image worthy of Constable. The horse carts were shaped like open-ended wooden feeding troughs. The driver sat on a simple plank in front of the trough and either passengers or material rode behind him. Drivers used two reins to control their horses but other horsemen also used horse whips to change the horse's direction when ploughing. The furrows they dug were perfectly straight. There are thousands of Lithuanian farmers who have not lost the rural art of horsemanship.

There were dead foxes on these roads—a more ominous sight here than in Western Europe.

Rabies is still endemic in Lithuania and is passed on to cattle through fox bites. Cattle account for well over half of all the confirmed cases of rabies in Lithuania each year.

Some fields here in the middle of the country extended to the far horizon, a physical reminder of Soviet collectivisation. The greater part of most of these fields had gone to seed and was covered by grassy meadow and scruffy shrubs, but scattered erratically within there were small cultivated patches, some of which had been harvested or soon would be. Some of these plots were potato patches, the plants were still green, and the potatoes now being harvested from them would have thin skins. These were for personal use, not for sale. Commercial potatoes need tougher skins and develop them if the plants above soil are killed a week or more before harvesting. I stopped frequently. Each town had an immaculately restored Catholic church in its centre. In Estonia the churches were set apart. Here they are central to life, physically and mentally.

Macy and I went for an hour-long walk in one of the variegated meadowy fields. In the distance, away from the sun, a huge raptor—I think it was a young golden eagle—sat in the field like a chocolate-brown scarecrow, then soared up and on its long, lazy wings flew into the adjacent pine woodlands. My dog didn't notice. She was preoccupied with meadow prey and incessantly performed two-paw cat pounces at them until I got bored and commanded her to move on. The land was boggy at the distant end of that field and naturally she bog-walked.

I showered the black bog muck off her and

continued to Kėdainiai, the pickle capital of the
Baltic—if I translated the sign correctly. On back
roads beyond Kėdainiai, I saw a sign saying
'Kauna'. I was now in the heart of 'Kovna
Gaberna', the region the Fogles and Bernards left
125 years ago.

There were seemingly as many dogs as horses in
this flat landscape. Wherever I stopped, dogs
barked. Whenever I walked past a home, tethered
dogs strained at their ropes or chains, desperate to
rip our gizzards out. Some were large dogs, but
more common, especially amongst those that
wandered freely along the highways, were small
dogs—around 10 kilograms in weight, with short
legs, erect ears and fox-like faces.

*   *   *

I passed more hay-filled carts being pulled by
horses and more haystacks. On the uncompleted
stacks the central poles were still visible. In one
field a woman in a headscarf was digging up beets.
In another, an older woman also wearing a
headscarf was drawing water from an outside well.
There were grey-brick farmhouses but more
frequently, box-shaped wooden homes. Some had
half-glassed front porches. This was a true peasant
land, much as it was imagined in family folk
memory.

While Estonia and Latvia were for ever
someone else's, Lithuania has its own history with
its own kings and nobility and even its own empire.
In *The Canterbury Tales*, Chaucer's Knight
mentions campaigning against the pagans in
'Samogitia' which is present-day Lithuania, for this

was the last region of Europe to convert to Christianity. The district of 'Samogitia' roughly corresponds to what my father called 'Kovna Gaberna' and, what was properly called 'Kovno Guberniya'. The Samogitian pagans didn't convert to Christianity until 1417.

Old traditions still endure. If you look carefully at the massed hordes of the Lithuanian crosses that have become twenty-first century tourist sites, they are not as Catholic as they seem. With their elaborately carved suns and moons these are pre-Christian pagan totems, adapted, just as the Christmas tree was adapted, to serve the new religion. There were medieval kings in Lithuania—Mindaugas, Gediminas, Vytautas—names that died and have arisen again with modern Lithuanian nationalism. After conversion to Christianity the aristocracy vacillated between Latin and Orthodox Christian options but in 1569 Lithuania fell on the Catholic side of the fence and formed a Union with Poland: the Polish-Lithuanian Commonwealth.

In the cosmopolitan 'Grand Duchy of Lithuania—Kingdom of Poland Commonwealth' six languages were officially recognised: Polish, German, Latin, Ruthene, (the language of present day Ukraine), Armenian and Hebrew. Eighty per cent of the world's Jews today trace their ancestry to this tolerant state. The Lithuanian language however, was not recognised. It was the language of the peasantry, and peasants played no part in law or commerce. Law was enacted in Latin and Polish while commerce was transacted in German, Ruthenian, Hebrew and Armenian.

The Polish-Lithuanian Commonwealth was in

the geographical centre of Europe's ongoing civil war between the Orthodox East and the Latin West. Prussia and Austria challenged the union from the west while Russia did so from the east. The region was partitioned and partitioned again. In the 'Third Partition' in 1795, both Poland and Lithuania ceased to exist. They were simply devoured by their challengers.

The whole of Lithuania came under Russian control and the Russians carried off Lithuania's state archives—every charter, act, statute and land deed they could find dating back to the Middle Ages. The country's history was comprehensively stolen. Some of this national archive was returned in 1921 but that was reappropriated by the Soviets in 1945. Since then the Russians have said there is no proof that what they hold in St. Petersburg had its origins in Lithuania but in the 1980s, an American scholar meticulously examining a catalogue made in seventeenth-century Warsaw by the invading Swedes, confirmed that the collection in St. Petersburg had its origins in Lithuania.

It can be difficult to know who you are if your identity has been stolen and the Lithuanians are solving their dilemma by creating a national mythology based upon ancient rural mythology. There's no room in that mythology for the fact that until very recently another large ethnic group made up a considerable part of the population of Lithuania. My ancestors were part of that group.

*　　　*　　　*

The mosquito-plagued campsite behind the information centre in Druskininkai had showers,

186

clothes' washing machines, a vehicle wash, electricity plug-ins, a level landscape and a 24-hour guard at the gate. I spent a couple of days in and around this spa town on the Nemunas River only a few kilometres from the Belarus border.

Druskininkai was a popular mud spa during the Soviet era and the massive buttresses of sanatoria the Soviets built still remain. The modern town is almost charming. The small, butterfly blue-and-white, clapboard, nineteenth-century, Russian Orthodox Church, with five purple-tiled domes and a taller central belfry was almost cartoon-like in its pristine prettiness—certainly the most attractive little church I saw in all of Lithuania.

Throughout the town there are expansive gingerbread wooden villas with elaborately carved eaves, windows, doors, verandas and pillars. Smaller wooden homes line the streets including one that was the home of the artist, Mikalojus Konstantinas Čiurlionis, and another where the artist Jacques Lipchitz lived. Both are museums.

It's a five-minute walk through pine woodlands from the campsite to the first of two lakes in town. The flowerbeds were immaculate, the riverside walk meticulously manicured and the buildings either repaired or still fit enough to be refurbished. I bought some local Druskininkai mineral water but could barely drink it, it tasted so slimy. I spared Macy its mineral excess and used it for washing dishes. The local spicy sausages were better. I sliced and fried them and had them with eggs for dinner.

At dusk Macy turned into a local dog, barking fiercely from her routine position resting on the ground outside the Roadtrek, while I cooked and

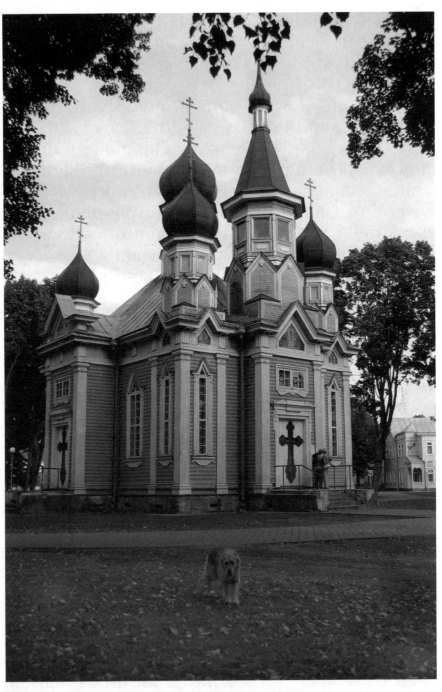

THE RUSSIAN ORTHODOX CHURCH AT
DRUSKININKAI

cowered inside, safe from the mosquito plague. I went out to see what had provoked her and saw a man nearby, with his bicycle turned broadside to protect himself from what he assumed was imminent attack.

'Sorry,' I said, *'Pardon, scusi.'* I hadn't a clue how to say 'sorry' in Lithuanian.

'Deutsch?' he smiled and his grip on the handlebars of his bike relaxed.

'English. *Angelski,'* I replied figuring that if you added '-ski' it made it sound Slavic.

'Medus?' he asked, and proffered a jar of honey.

Medus. Mead! It sounded familiar. In his shoulder-bag were jars of honey and in entrepreneurial new Lithuania he was visiting the only inhabitant of the only campsite in town hoping to make a sale. Of course he did. After buying honey by chance in Holland and then from the roadside stand in Denmark and then from a local bee-keeper on Gotland I'd been bitten by the honey bug and had intentionally bought a pot in every successive country, from shops in Finland and Latvia and from a roadside honey-seller in Estonia.

This man's tawny-coloured set honey had been squashed into unlabelled glass jars. It was mild in its sweetness, perfect in the last of the fresh mint tea I brewed from the plants I'd picked in Estonia.

In my planning for this trip I'd made contact with a Lithuanian veterinarian and he'd suggested visiting a bee museum in the north of the country near where he lived. He'd explained in emails that bees and honey had special significance in Lithuania. An old word for especially close friends was *'biciuliai'* or 'bee friends'. Honey was

189

associated with fertility, hard work, loyalty, decency.

Historically it had not been part of the money economy but rather was given to beggars at Christmas, to friends and neighbours on special occasions, after a woman gave birth or to help celebrate festive occasions. To Lithuanians, he wrote, sharing honey, especially between relatives and close friends was an act of great ritual significance. That's a tradition I was raised in too—the sharing between family, friends, even passing strangers in need of food, of apples dipped in honey at Passover.

*   *   *

The surrounding sandy soiled, dense, pine forest with its occasional exposed areas of virtual sand dune was curiously similar in look and aroma to the pine woodlands of De Hoge Veluwe in Holland. It even had countless bicycle paths although I failed to meet people on them. I didn't go out of my way to meet anyone, and the locals didn't either.

North-east of Druskininkai in rolling countryside, farming was more mechanised than it was further west. Here, women drove across the fields and parked their cars beside their cows when they milked them. South-east to the Belarus border there was only tall pine forest but in that forest, at the end of a twisting road through the ramshackle wooden village of Grūtaas is Grūto Parkas, Stalin World to headline writers. That's where I was headed.

I parked the Roadtrek by a vintage cattle car,

bought my ticket and to the sound of Soviet martial music from speakers high in the surrounding trees walked the 30 hectare site. I was its only visitor. There's a zoo, of sorts, with small wire-runs housing various breeds of ornamental chickens, a children's playground, a café, a couple of fierce-looking crop-eared Dobermanns on thick leads being walked by black-clad thugs—the park's security—and a two-kilometre figure-eight wooden walkway through woodlands, lined with icons of the Soviet era, 86 statues once meant to provoke worship and respect for the Communist Party.

At the beginning of the walk, as you round a bend to the left there are 13 Lenins, including one seated with his legs crossed and his left hand on a book. I sat on his lap. Until 1990 it adorned the main square in Druskinkinkai and until 1990 if I'd sat on his lap I'd have ended up detained as a 'patient' in a psychiatric hospital. Another Lenin, with an outstretched right arm, used to face the KGB building in Vilnius. There's only one statue of Stalin at Stalin World, which is not surprising as Khrushchev ordered most of them to be removed and melted down.

Many of the other statues were of Lithuanian Communists. Zigmas Angarietis, a graduate of the Warsaw Veterinary Institute, was the first People's Commissar of Internal Affairs of the Lithuanian Soviet Socialist Republic and, the inscription told me, had implemented the terror policy in 1918. Stalin had him arrested in 1938 during one of his regular Communist Party cleansings and he died in prison in 1940. There's a 47-ton copper statue, welded together in Minsk, of eight cone-shaped freedom fighters—broad-based figures with tiny

191

heads. When it was first loaded for transport to Grūtaas the truck's 16 tyres all popped like blisters.

The most intriguing—if only because it looked like a bunch of drunks, not idealised Communists—was one of four angry young men, Pozela, Greifenbergeris, Carnas and Gyederys. Gyederys eventually emigrated to Arlington, Massachusetts where he set up a Boston branch of the Communist Party. The English translation posted beside the statue didn't explain what the others did, nor was there a reason given for why they deserved their own statue. I assume they were young revolutionaries but the statues make them look more like hooligans. Then again, what's the difference between so many 'revolutionaries' and street thugs?

The statues are here because, after destroying some and selling others to metal traders or to Western collectors, the Lithuanian government put them in warehouses and yards owned by newly privatised utility companies. Storage was costing money and to offset that cost an auction was held for the right to display the remaining statues. All the bidders' proposals but one included the assumption that the annual running costs would be paid by the government. The offer by a local mushroom magnate to do it himself appealed to cash-strapped politicians and Viliumas Malinauskas built Grūto Parkas to house them.

Back at the ticket kiosk I asked if I could take Macy inside to take pictures of her. After several long telephone calls the answer was 'no'. I explained that I was a journalist and wanted to take a photo of Macy peeing on Lenin's leg but they failed to see the irony and I was firmly told that regulations stated dogs were not permitted in the park. No exceptions.

*　　　*　　　*

I was looking for a shortcut to the hamlet of Margionys in the heart of Dzūkijos National Park when I chanced upon a ten-kilometre long sandy tract through tinder-dry pine forest. Off the main road I had passed through a village of peasant farmsteads, each with apple trees, chickens, tethered dogs, piles of firewood and unending junk, heaped behind unpainted wooden fences. Cows, including one that was the mushroom colour of a Weimaraner, were tethered, either beside each home or within the surrounding fence. As I drove I saw a golden-orange bird of prey twice the size of a kestrel gliding solemnly over the surrounding meadowland.

Beyond the village was forest and the local map I'd picked up in Druskinkinkai showed a road through it. What I hadn't noticed was that the thickness of the line on the map marking this road was considerably less than the thickness of others, and it was only after I had been bouncing along it for several miles, spinning the wheels in drifts of sand in the dips, scraping the sides of the Roadtrek against vegetation on both sides, whipping the aerial on passing branches, that I realised there were no tyre tracks on it. I was the first vehicle to use it for ages.

Around half an hour down the track I stopped. There was nowhere to pull off and park but I didn't need to: I was in deep nothingness, surely one of the most isolated regions of the entire country. It was serenely beautiful, a light sunny landscape of tall pines. The ground was covered in purple flowering heathers, red lingonberries, pale white, red and green mosses, twigs, fallen branches and endless mushrooms. I couldn't identify most of them but I did recognise chanterelles.

In 1982 I was invited to a dinner in Vienna honouring Konrad Lorenz, the Nobel Prize-winning ethologist. At that meal Lorenz said that it was only luck and good fortune that led to his being awarded the Nobel Prize for his work in animal behaviour, and his research on maternal imprinting behaviour in greyleg geese. 'Ideas,' he said 'spread like fungal mycelia beneath the surface of the forest floor. Mushrooms erupt from the ground and they appear unique but they are not. Like one of those mushrooms my ideas seemed original, but hidden beneath the surface it was connected to others, now forgotten. I was the right mushroom in the right place at the right time.'

As I picked chanterelles from the Dzūkijos forest floor I wondered how far their mycelia spread. A metre? Five metres? Fifty metres? Mycelia can live for one hundred, three hundred, even six hundred years. Mushrooms hundreds of metres apart in this woods could be genetic clones. My dinner tonight could have been alive and living here in this forest 300 years ago when my great-great-great-great-great-great-grandfather was living less than 100 kilometres away.

This land is so remote and so infertile that World War Two passed it by. Even Soviet era collectivisation mostly bypassed these woods. The isolated farmsteads and fields deep in the forest retain their ancient patterns. These hidden villages or *'shtetls'* as they were called in Russian and Yiddish, are all that remain of traditional rural Lithuanian life as it was lived before 1918.

In that year all estates over 80 hectare were nationalised. Their collections, valuables and libraries were dispersed. In Soviet times the remaining smallholdings were collectivised. Fields were enlarged to accommodate massive combine harvesters. Marshes were drained. The courses of streams changed. Land was reclaimed and life in rivers and lakes was altered by run-off from chemicals used to fertilise agricultural lands. The focus of rural life was destroyed. These few hidden villages are now rightly called 'ethno-cultural reserves'.

Margionys was magic. The Soviets had been here and there were occasional rectangular grey-brick monstrosities but the oldest homes, built of square-cut interlocked logs, remained. Newer ones, probably built at the turn of the twentieth century were rectangular, clapboard-sided with porches on the long side and shutters on the windows. Some had never been painted while others were the traditional mustard yellow and brown of the region. Each was surrounded by an unpainted wooden picket fence. Several homes had collections of beehives in their apple tree gardens. The beehives were all a similar shape, like Georgian doll's houses, painted mustard yellow, brown or pale sky blue. The brown hives had white triangles painted above the bees' entry platforms.

The freshly restored wooden church at isolated

Kapeliai has two steeples and a separate bell tower on the church grounds, much like the church in Saaremaa. I was going to take Macy for a long walk after visiting it but I was less than a kilometre from the Belarus border and got worried that she might choose to make an illicit crossing so I took the dirt road to the village of Mustieka a few kilometres away.

There were beehives here too, some made out of hollow logs, and, as everywhere else, barking dogs at each homestead we walked past. A track led south from Mustieka, through open fields and then woods and I took that past a giant stork's nest perched precariously on a barn. From the day the Russians arrived, and then the Germans after them, partisans took to these forests: Lithuanian, Belarusian, Polish, Jewish, Bolshevik. Some were still there until the 1950s, some until the 1960s. The last of the Baltic's 'Forest Brothers' died escaping capture in 1974.

Macy raised a brace of wood grouse then became preoccupied with a scent she picked up. She sniffed the ground then inhaled from a tree than sniffed another part of the ground that had been disturbed. There were animal droppings, dark, like fox droppings but larger. It looked like fresh dog turds but this dog had not eaten roughage. Macy had picked up wolf scent. I reined her in and we continued but as the roadside became boggier I turned and retreated to the Roadtrek, taking her back to green fields where she rolled, surrounded by white butterflies. In the absence of wolves to chase she entertained herself chasing wagtails.

At a junction with the paved road to the large

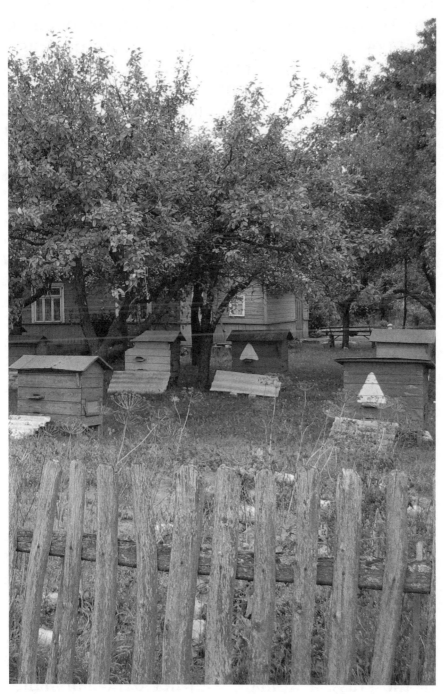

Doll's house beehives at Margionys

village of Marcinkonys I picked up a couple of middle-aged, local hitchhikers. He, unkempt, in dust-covered clothing, sat in the front passenger seat while she, tidier, more dignified, took the back seat. We drove silently past a collection of austere, abandoned grey-brick buildings—probably an old collective farm—and crisp, new, Dzūkijos National Park's buildings beside it.

We passed a family of seven collecting potatoes from a small patch of land reclaimed from a vast field that had otherwise gone to seed. There were churns by the roadside and an old *babushka* walking along the side of the road with a sack of potatoes on her back. I had questions I wanted to ask my passengers but the language barrier was frustratingly overwhelming. At Marcinkonys, grinning a gold-toothed smile, my passenger proffered a four litas payment for the ride. His wife, sitting in the back, stroked Macy for the entire journey.

* * *

There is a collection of old farmsteads at a crossroad at Trasnykas. The buildings, including the houses, are constructed of the characteristic interlocking logs and the doors, both to the barns and the homes, are ornamented with multiple criss-crossing patterns in wood. They looked as if a carpenter had carried out cross-stitching on them. I stopped to photograph these intricate designs and while I was doing so, and as Macy was rolling in the grass, a woman, with her dark hair pulled back in a bun, wearing a faded, striped blue wool jacket over a blue on blue striped jumper, came

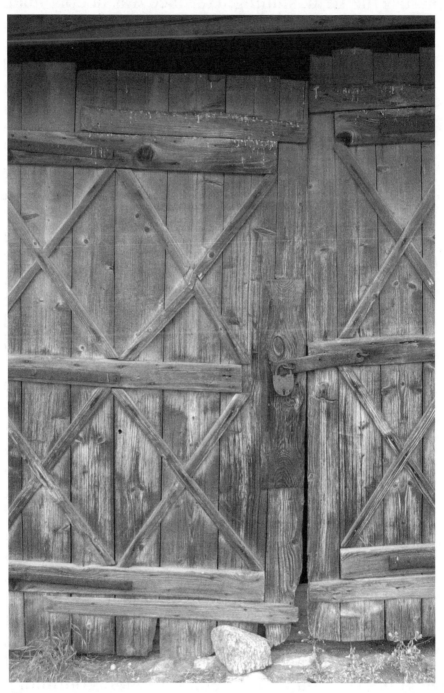

CROSS-STITCHED BARN DOORS AT TRASNYKAS

across the field, smiling. Her face was deeply lined as if it were formed from artist's clay.

'*Labas. Laba diena. Vokiškai?*'

I knew the first two words, 'Hello. Good afternoon.' but didn't know '*Vokiškai*' meant 'German' until it was explained to me the next day.

I replied with my 'sorry' routine.

'*Angliskai!*' she exclaimed, triumphant. Now her neighbour, older, plumper, also with her dark hair pulled back in a bun, joined her, listening but seldom speaking.

The woman carried on a one-sided 15-minute conversation with me and didn't stop once for breath until I asked, by raising my camera, if I could take her picture. Her hand language explained that she wasn't prepared for a photo and wanted to tidy herself up, but then she relented and I took a few photos of the two women petting Macy. Then, with head and arm movements she directed me towards her home, a rusting tin-roofed building behind an unpainted picket fence.

I hesitated, not because I didn't want to follow her. Her Rottweiler had been silently watching from behind the wooden fence and I don't trust silent Rotties. She opened the gate and beckoned us in and I put Macy on her lead and followed. The Rottweiler, attached to its dog house by a thick rope, just watched.

Inside I was offered firewater in an etched glass, a distillation she must have made herself that tasted like turpentine mixed with antifreeze. I was given black bread and a bowl of cold cabbage and lingonberry soup. I listened to her continuing monologue, regretted not understanding a word of it, but questioned what cynical Andreas had told me in London: 'The country people. They are very suspicious. You are better to visit the cities.'

Heavy rain came and the sound of drops bouncing off the tin roof of her home almost drowned out her story. The industrial meths she shared with me made me see double Roadtreks when I left but I successfully made my way past her Rottweiler back to my vehicle and departed.

'*Iki!*' she waved, '*Iki!*' 'Bye bye'. The rain was cold and biting. Summer was broken. A frigid wind followed. It would be cold in Kaunas.

*   *   *

Two other campers had joined me in Druskininkai that night, both German, and both with dogs, a young yellow Labrador and a rough lurcher type. The Labrador spent the next morning sitting still on the passenger seat of his motorhome, a keen observer of Europe, while the lurcher gambolled with Macy. Getting back from our morning walk I noticed I'd lost the metal guard to the exterior access pipe for the hot water unit to the Roadtrek the previous day. It must have been ripped off by branches as I drove along the unused sandy tract through Dzūkijos forest.

CABBAGE AND LINGONBERRY SOUP
On a dry day pick 200g of carmine-coloured lingonberries.
Harvest, clean and slice 400g of white cabbage.
Boil the lingonberries just until they burst then strain them through a sieve to remove forest floor debris.
Place the cabbage in a litre of water, add the

sieved lingonberries and gently cook until the cabbage is tender.
Remove from heat and thicken with two beaten eggs and 100g of cream.
Season with salt, pepper, lemon juice and, if it's too tart for your taste, a little brown sugar.

*   *   *

When he was well into his nineties I gave my father a list of questions and a small tape recorder and asked him to record his memories, just for the sake of giving him something to do on rainy days during what turned out to be his last winter in Sarasota, Florida. The list started with simple questions. Where did you grow up? 'Britannia Heights'. What did people call your father? 'JR.' Why did the Fogles leave Kovna? 'The Cossacks.'

Plausible, but I don't know if this is true. During my weekly childhood violin lessons from my father's older brother, Myer, who played viola in the Toronto Symphony Orchestra, I once asked the same question and he told me his grandfather smuggled tobacco across the Prussian border. One day his 'tame' border guard told him there was to be a major offensive against smugglers and my great-grandfather took his family, including his young sons Jacob and Philip, caught a boat and moved elsewhere, as it happens, to Glasgow. When he arrived there the Jewish community was small—less than a thousand—jute and wool merchants, quill and fruit merchants, furriers, watchmakers, saloonkeepers. By the time his son moved on to Canada, 25 years later, the population had increased almost eightfold, mostly

202

from Lithuania.

Whatever the reason they left, I was back on the E67, now a wide motorway, driving to Kovno—now called Kaunas. On the radio what sounded like more dire Eurovision Song Contest auditions were taking place and as I listened a guy in a car in front of me came to a complete stop on the road, deciding whether or not to take the motorway exit. And his tail-lights weren't working. I was seven tons of mass hurtling up his tailpipe but through sheer good fortune I didn't become the first Fogle to die here in 125 years. Macy was not amused by the emergency stop and after she regained her composure she crawled under my legs for added security.

The motorway's road surface was excellent but as soon as I left it and headed into the city I was back on rolling, bumpy, potholed roads typical of virtually everywhere I'd travelled in the Baltic states. Nine-storey, anonymous, grey-bricked, Soviet apartment blocks sprouted from the surrounding fields like dusty rectangular mushrooms. Trolley buses busily worked the roads, their drivers separated from the passengers by pull-down, patterned curtains. Innumerable private minivans were also busy working the street, picking up passengers from bus-stops. The sky was muddy. Dank clouds wrapped the dire towers. It was all depressing.

*   *   *

I found the Neris hotel where I had arranged to meet a local man, Simonas Dovidavicius, and bought eight hours of parking meter time from the local police station. I got a telephone call from Simonas telling me he'd be late and walked the streets for an hour. It was grim. We walked the nearby wide, pedestrianised, nineteenth-century shopping boulevard but even the flower seller with her multitude of plastic buckets of gladioli was colourless. The mock-Byzantine St. Michael's Church, once Orthodox, an art gallery during Soviet times, now Catholic, sat broodily like a scarab beetle at the eastern end of the mall.

Simonas cheered me up. He was dishevelled, rotund, always smiling, ready to embrace you. 'Bruce, I'm so sorry. Business,' he grinned as he shook my hand with one of his and grasped my shoulder with the other. One shirt-tail hung out from his trousers. Good humour scintillated from his warm blue eyes. Simonas took me to Sugihara House, a private museum, where he is curator, and had to attend to some still unfinished business.

Chiune Sugihara's story is not well known but is a compelling, remarkable and ennobling one. Born in Japan to a middle-class mother and a samurai-class father, he studied English at university, joined the Japanese Foreign Ministry and became an expert on Russian Affairs. In 1939 he was posted by his government as vice-consul of the Japanese Consulate in Kaunas. His remit was to report on Soviet and German troop movements.

When the Soviets took over Lithuania in 1940, many Polish Jewish refugees who had fled there from the invading Germans the year previously, tried to leave. The Dutch consul Jan Zwartendijk helped, providing paperwork for entry to Curaçao and Dutch Guyana in the Caribbean and South America. Sugihara asked his superiors in Tokyo

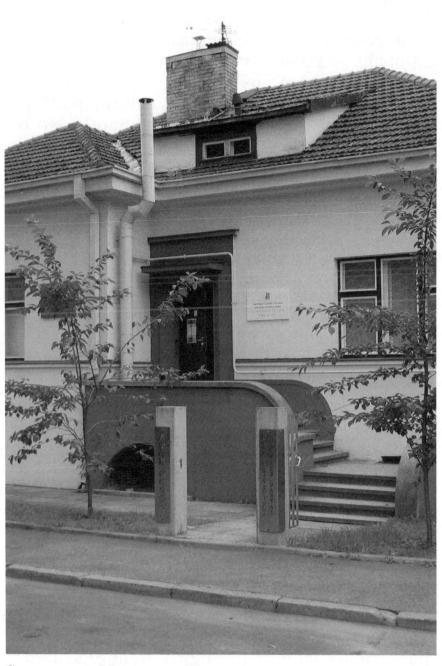

Sugihara House in Kaunas

for permission to issue transit visas through Japan but was refused. He asked on two more occasions but was told that Japanese immigration guidelines must be followed. The Polish refugees living in Lithuania could not meet these criteria.

In violation of his orders and, to me, more astonishingly, in violation of his culture, he started issuing transit visas on his own initiative. No one knows exactly how many of these handwritten documents he issued but it was certainly in the thousands. He spoke to Soviet officials and got their agreement for his visa holders to travel, on payment of a 500 per cent surcharge, via the Trans-Siberian railway, across Asia to Kobe, in Japan.

Some remained there, some were deported for the duration of the war to Japanese-occupied Shanghai and some made their way to the United States, Canada and the British Mandate of Palestine. Twenty-eight years later, one of the children who he helped escape, Joshua Nishri, was posted by his government as economic attaché to the Israeli Embassy in Tokyo. Nishri sought out Sugihara and discovered that after Kaunas he had been assigned by his government to Prague, then Bucharest. When Romania fell to the Russians he was imprisoned by the Soviets for 18 months and on his release in 1946 returned to Japan via the Trans-Siberian railway. In 1947 the Japanese Foreign Office asked him to resign.

Nishri invited Sugihara, the man who saved his family, to visit Israel and his story became known there. Years later that country honoured him as one of the 'Righteous Amongst the Nations', the highest honour Israel can bestow.

When he told me this tale, Simonas explained that all stories, even the most appealing, are based on selective memory. It is likely, he explained, that it was Mrs Sugihara who suggested to her husband that he issue transit visas. It is also likely that the first visas were issued to Jewish families fleeing the Soviets and only latterly to those fleeing the Germans. All the photos in the museum—of refugees at the gate of the legation or later on a boat bound from Shanghai for Canada—show highly educated, well-dressed people. These people were from the same social class, the same caste, as Sugihara. When asked why he did what he did he simply answered that these people were human beings who needed help.

The museum is a shoestring affair. The guest chairs in Simonas' maelstrom of an office were two, well-worn front car seats. While a coach load of Japanese tourists descended from their bus, the museum tour guide, another Ohio-sized woman in her forties, proudly showed me photographs of her European laika.

I asked Simonas why he set up Sugihara House and he told me that his grandmother and mother had been saved by Lithuanian Sugiharas, by a farming family near Klaipėda, who told the authorities that the women, the girl and her young mother, were relatives. Simonas' daily work takes him into the cold heart and reality of recent Lithuanian history but he doesn't think it unusual that his mother and grandmother were saved by the farmers. He considers their action 'normal': what any moral person would do. Simonas sees inherent goodness in people.

I asked how many Jews now lived in Lithuania—

at the time of the Third Partition, in 1793 there were around 250,000, a quarter of the entire population. Simonas answered, '4007'.

I'd been put in touch with Simonas through a vet in London and was in Kaunas to try to find where the Fogles and Bernards once lived. I was familiar with the basics. The first stream of Jewish immigrants arrived in Lithuania in the 800s from the east, from the Caucasus and southern Russia. Another stream arrived later from the west, from England where they had been expelled in 1215, from France and from Germany—families escaping to the east to get away from the Crusaders.

They were joined 300 years later by a third group, Spanish and Portuguese Jews expelled by the Inquisition from their homes on the Iberian peninsula in 1492. The Spanish and Portuguese families had different proper names, pronounced Yiddish in different ways, even looked different and had not completely blended in with the rest of the population until the eighteenth century.

I knew my ancestors were '*Litvaks*' but didn't know exactly what the word meant. Simonas explained it simply meant people from the region the Jews called 'Lita' or 'Lithuania' composed of present day western Belarus, all of Lithuania, bits of Latvia and small parts of northern Poland.

'You know, at the 1919 Versailles Peace Conference, the Lithuanian delegate joked that what he would like for his country is everything the Jews called Lithuania.'

'The word "*Litvak*" is also associated with Haskala and the Enlightenment,' he explained, 'with a questioning style of teaching. Hasidism and

Cabbalism never took hold with Litvaks. Those teachings were more prevalent amongst Polish and Galician Jews.'

'Any luck, finding where the Fogles and Bernards might have lived?' I asked, because I'd been in contact with Simonas before I left London and had explained what I was looking for. He told me he was no genealogist but there was a problem because 'Kovno Guberniya' was such a large region. He hit the government website on his computer, printed out a detailed map and then asked, 'Do you have the name of an *uyezd* or *shtetl*?'

Each *guberniya* was divided into districts or '*uyezds*'. Kovno Guberniya had seven districts in it. In front of him were lists of all villages, towns and cities in present-day Lithuania, giving their modern names and their old Russian or Yiddish village or '*shtetl*' names. Beside each village name was the name of the local district, the '*uyezd*' and the larger province, the '*guberniya*'.

I asked exactly how large Kovno province was and, cross-referencing from his list he started marking the map. When he finished both he and I learned that Kovno Guberniya extended from the Baltic coastline in the west, up to and along the Latvia border to the Belarus border to the east, down just to the east of Kaunas to the next *guberniya*, Suwalki to the south, and along the border of the Russian Kaliningrad enclave, old East Prussia, back to the Baltic. It covered over 90 per cent of modern Lithuania.

'Without more information I'm afraid it's not possible to know where your families lived.'

I looked closely at the detailed map of the

country and saw that the Nemunas River separates old East Prussia from Kovno Guberniya. Perhaps my Uncle Myer's smuggling story had substance.

*   *   *

My surname wasn't much help. It's German and simply means 'bird' and gives no clues to its origins. Before 1793 all Jewish names were patronymics. This is true of Scandinavian surnames as well, and there patronymics became fixed around the same time. My Swedish friends Lars Gustafsson and Johan Nilsson are not the sons of Gustaf and Nils but both of those were the given names of their male ancestors at the time their surnames were fixed. In that sense my patronymic name in English would be Bruce Morrisson, as Morris was my dad's name. In Hebrew his name was Moshe and mine Baruch, so pre-1793 I'd have been Baruch ben Moshe.

Napoleon put an end to that when he declared that henceforth all Jews must adopt modern European names. In Prussia and Austria, Jews were usually allotted German names by state officials. Some names such as Goldstein, Rubenstein and Silverstein were given by officials who believed Jews had precious stones hidden in their homes. After the Partition of Poland and Lithuania, when Warsaw was Prussian-occupied, that city's chief Prussian administrator from 1795 to 1806, ETA Hoffmann, selected surnames according to his whim: Vogel, Vogelsang, Apfelbaum, Himmelfarb, or less attractively, Fischgrund, Fischbein or Katzenellenbogen.

As was common in Germany and England,

many families took on the names of their trades. Shoemakers took the name Schuster, tailors took Schneider while carpenters became Tischler. Some chose or were given names from nature, Rosenberg—mountain of roses, Lilienthal—valley of the lilies, Schonberg—beautiful mountain. In French, Schonbergs became Belmonts. Others adopted the names of the towns or cities they lived in: Oppenheimer, Frankfurter, Pressburger.

Jewish emancipation and the acquisition of new names was double-edged. My ancestors had to escape from the internal ghetto in their minds too. This demanded the reconciliation of the principles of their faith with the demands of an emerging modern society. Some found that more straightforward than others and it was easier in Lithuania under the influence of *Haskala*—the Jewish Enlightenment—than it was in regions of Europe where Cabbalistic mysticism had captured minds. For people raised in the Jewish cultural traditions in Lithuania and in the German-speaking regions of Europe, where it was accepted, even demanded of them to ask questions and have open minds, opportunities were unprecedented and led to their formidable contributions to twentieth century European culture and achievement.

In a restaurant on top of a skyscraper in Tokyo I once asked a psychiatrist acquaintance, Aaron Katcher, why it was that in a field as obscure as people–pet relations—which we were in Japan to discuss—so many of the scholars or commentators such as himself, Boris Levinson, Alan Beck, Sam Corson, and myself were Jewish. He suggested that it was not just because we had a common upbringing in a culture with a passion for education or philosophical argument. For people in a psychological limbo between one culture and another there is also a determination to search for the new, and to overcome rejection. The reason why, for example, 47 per cent of Viennese doctors or 62 per cent of Viennese lawyers in 1936 were Jewish, or why for the first half of the twentieth century in Europe Jews were the prime patrons or participants in new art, architecture, music, science, philosophy, the avant-garde, was that having 'turned their backs' on their old culture they were positively disposed to the challenging and the new.

I concluded that my surname would be of no value in looking for historic ancestors but Simonas explained that this was not necessarily so.

'There are Russian Revision Lists, *Reviskie Skazkie*, from the early 1800s that might bridge the gap between your present name and your family's former names. A genealogist who reads Polish and Russian is needed. I can put you in touch with such a person. He might find "Fogle" in one of these Russian lists. Before that, the tax lists are written in Polish in the Latin alphabet. There are also estate inventories in Polish from the same period. The nobility lived on their estates and farms but commerce and industry was managed for them by Jewish leaseholders. The Jews collected rent for them. I have a copy—just given to me—of an inventory for Ukmergė. Ukmergė is about 75 kilometres from here,' and he rummaged in his piles of books and papers and miraculously found it.

'An American Jew I took on a Holocaust tour

sent it to me.' Simonas showed me a thick bundle of papers printed off the Internet with handwritten annotations in the margins.

'It is very interesting. 1773. Vilkomir. It shows Jews rented particular meadows. They sold hay and had vegetable gardens. They leased mills and breweries and inns from the noblemen. The Russian Revision Lists from the early 1800s are of course in Russian. These include the Jews' modern surnames. The Russians used these lists for conscripting quotas of Jewish boys into the Tsar's army—for 15 years. Jewish mothers were the same then. They lied about their children so they would not be conscripted. Some families rushed their boys into marriage before they reached puberty. Birth dates were altered. Bribes offered. The brunt of the edict fell on orphans and children of the poor. Child catchers were employed to steal children from other villages.'

The Muslim and Jewish graves I visited amongst the lingonberries and birch trees on Åland were doubtlessly those of conscript soldiers, whose mothers' lies had been disregarded.

Simonas is a local tour guide and asked me what type of tour I'd like, 'City tour, Jewish tour, Holocaust tour?' As it was the subject of the day I opted for 'Jewish Kaunas' and, in a car that was as gloriously dishevelled as he was, Simonas guided me through town, past the old Jewish hospital now derelict, past Jewish schools that were now state gymnasia, past the sole remaining synagogue and the old Jewish area of Svobodka where one of the rustic old wooden homes is now a veterinary pharmacy. At a Statoil station where we stopped for petrol he explained that he only buys gas from

Statoil. 'I'm a capitalist. I'm not interested in helping the Russian state by buying from Lukoil.'

Driving out to the Russian Ninth Fort, I told him where I'd travelled during my first few days in Lithuania. When I mentioned I'd been to the pickle capital of the Baltic he told me that Kėdainiai was more than that—it was a centuries-old centre of religious tolerance. 'There are many Scottish names in Kėdainiai. Over 3000 Scottish people—Calvinists—settled there to escape religious persecution in Scotland. It was a very learned city. Many printing houses. Before the war almost 10 per cent of the Jewish families were involved in the pickle trade. They employed hundreds.'

A large local population of Scots could explain why my Californian cousin Erik has a genetic heritage that connects him to Strathclyde, Scotland. As well as mercenaries and merchants, the Scots were also unexpected migrants to the east. A part of the family jigsaw fell into place.

I asked how it was that the Lithuanians turned on their Jewish neighbours. He had told me, as we drove through Svobodka, that local people killed 2000 of their neighbours before the Germans arrived.

'Cultural suspicion is universal: the stereotype of the sharp-witted city-dweller and the dim-witted farmer. There was always some anti-Semitism in peasant tradition, and businessmen were jealous of the success of the Jews but it is more complicated than that.

'Jewish irony is completely alien to Lithuanian tradition. Just as for years New York Jewish humour was only understood by Jews, it caused distrust. Rural people didn't understand it. It was garlic to vampires. Of course this is different now, but it was impossible for Lithuanians to understand Jews, to understand you can have allegiance to the country you live in without being an ethnic Lithuanian. It is still hard for some to understand.

'When the Lithuanian language was developing and a national literature written, Jews did not participate. The language had few attractions. German, Polish, especially Russian, these languages were a passport to the world, not Lithuanian. The Russian world was cosmopolitan and willing to accept foreigners who used their language so well. Jewish Lithuanians were drawn to Russia. The Russian intelligentsia opposed the Tsar and the result was that educated Lithuanian Jews were leftists. They knew what was happening in German-occupied lands and when the Russians invaded many Jews welcomed them.

'The Soviets gave these Jews visibility and now the Lithuanians thought "all the Soviets are Jews". The truth is that proportionally Stalin deported twice as many Jewish Lithuanians as Christian Lithuanians to the gulag. Lithuanians forgot that the Russians exiled the entire Jewish community to Russia in World War One when they thought that because they shared a common language they might aid the Germans. It is so complicated.'

It was cold, not much more than 10°C when we parked at the Kaunas Fortress. An oppressive dank mist clung to the landscape. The massive forts surrounding Kaunas were built at the end of the nineteenth and beginning of the twentieth centuries by the Tsar to defend this distant outpost

215

of the Empire from Germany. They were state-of-the-art defences, a series of fortresses placed around the city, 2–2.5 kilometres apart from each other and functioning almost like a single super fortress, with batteries plugging the gaps between them.

Each is set on high land above the roads and railway lines leading into Kaunas. The defensive ring around the city is completed by the Nemunas river to the south. Within the ring of forts was a military train station, government laboratories, military warehouses and workshops. Before the original eight forts were completed, 12 additional ones were planned, but only the ninth was completed to the architect's plan. In World War One, the Germans overran the forts' defences in 11 days. In World War Two, the Germans returned, this time bringing thousands of people here to murder them.

I know enough about this nadir in European history and didn't want to be revolted or sickened, or 'entertained' by stories of atrocities but I dutifully followed Simonas through the Ninth Fort Museum. He explained events and recited numbers, but I wasn't listening. I didn't want to listen. Then something caught my eye. People shipped here had written graffiti on the walls, graffiti now sanctified by panes of shatterproof glass.

Most was unintelligible to me but a simple sentence stood out, as if written in blood. *'Nous sommes 500 Français de Limoges.'* 'We are 500 Frenchmen from Limoges.'

In any other context it would have been the most banal of statements. 'We are 500 Frenchmen

216

from Limoges.' Limoges. The heart of France. Where Richard Lionheart was killed by a crossbow bolt in 1199. Where Pierre-Auguste Renoir was born. Where the most exquisitely beautiful porcelain ever created comes from. Did these men work in copper? In enamel? In porcelain? What were the occupations of these 500 Frenchmen, transported to this grim and distant fortress to be murdered simply because, as well as being Frenchmen from Limoges, they were Jewish Frenchmen? I felt like I'd been punched in the stomach. Such a simple statement. I had to leave.

Two years ago one of my patients, an emaciated 19-year-old brown Burmese cat, reached terminal decline. I discussed what we should do and the cat's owner, a beautiful, quiet and composed, elegant, gentle-eyed woman in her late eighties, agreed that her elderly friend should be euthanised. She asked if she could stay during the process. I prepared a small syringe of concentrated anaesthetic and as she stood and watched I injected it in a vein.

'Thank you,' she said and looked at her cat's dead body. 'It was so peaceful,' she added and she unclasped her mottled hands and gently stroked her cat's head and body.

Clear-eyed, she turned to me and thanked me again then added, 'This is the first time I have been with a member of my family when she died. I will be for ever grateful to you for that.' All of Mrs Weiss's family were killed in places like the Kaunas Ninth Fort. Only she survived.

*   *   *

217

A short distance east of Kaunas, just beyond the far end of Kaunas Lake, there is an expansive open-air rural heritage museum with a large parking lot where campers are permitted to park overnight. I headed there and woke the following morning to blue skies and autumn freshness. At dusk, two cars filled with local hunters had joined me. They donned their fatigues and armed with crossbows and aluminium arrows, spent the night doing what guys around the world seem to feel compelled to do. I'm glad to say they came back empty-handed.

This ethnographic museum is superb: 175 hectares, 140 buildings, 7 kilometres of one-way roads. I spent most of the day there. It's divided into four sections representing each quarter of the country. Dzūkijos is the only region of the countryside where I had lingered and the Dzūkijos sector of the museum was an accurate, if idealised, representation of it.

While flowers coloured the gardens in the museum, I hadn't seen a single blossom in the depths of Dzūkijos. And while buildings on display were thatch-roofed, in Dzūkijos proper they were invariably roofed in rusting tin. As in Skansen, the Swedish open-air museum in Stockholm, the homes were filled with rustic, often painted, furniture. The colours used and some of the floral styles too were similar to Scandinavian painted furniture but the cabinetry was rough and ill-finished. The furniture was prosaic, heavy, indelicate.

A school party was visiting the Suvalkija section and nibbles had been laid out for them—an assortment of thinly sliced sausages, salamis and

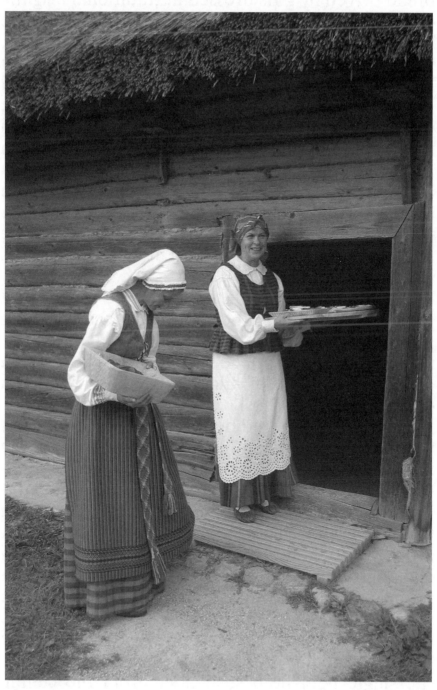

TRADITIONAL DRESS AT THE RURAL HERITAGE
MUSEUM NEAR KAUNAS

bread served by girls dressed in traditional brightly coloured embroidered dresses and headscarves. The nibbles were good. There were red apples too, soft and bruised but sweetly aromatic. In a building on the main street of the typical nineteenth-century town, amber workers, weavers, wood workers, jewellers and ceramists displayed their skills and sold their wares. I wanted to buy an attractive souvenir but the embroidery was garish and the weavings were only of King Vytautas in armour on his charging horse. The old *babushka* working the loom, wearing traditional dress and headscarf, scowled and barked at the giggling girls who milled around her.

A zillion sparrows flitted from tree to tree as I took Macy for an illicit walk on the museum grounds. I chanced on a damson tree, all of its fruit fallen during the previous day's rain storm, and collected a couple of kilos that had not yet been feasted upon by wasps.

Cows were tethered by chains on the grounds of the museum and when I left and drove through the adjacent town of Rumsiskes they were tethered there too, in fields between homes, even on front lawns. I chanced on a *'Veterinarijos Vaistiné'*, a veterinary pharmacy, an asbestos-roofed but attractive-looking, wooden, lime-green painted clapboard house with a large double-doored front porch. I walked through the porch into a side room where the walls and ceiling were made of the same tongue and groove 10 centimetre-wide brown painted panelling. A conical plastic shade wrapped the single light bulb suspended from the ceiling and behind a wooden, glass-fronted cabinet filled with rat poisons and flea treatments sat the chemist. He spoke no English. I bought a souvenir of Lithuania: more Frontline tick repellent for Macy.

DAMSONS IN SOUR CREAM
Halve around 500g of damson plums, remove the stones and make absolutely sure your dog doesn't eat the stones.
Put the plums in a deep bowl (suitable for use in the microwave) and add two tablespoons of 'Nemunas Midaus Nektaras'. This Lithuanian tipple claims to be 'Mead Nectar' but don't be fooled, as I was, and think that it is made from fermented honey. It's really 'Extra kind, grain ethyl alcohol and half-finished mead product', according to the fine print.
Sprinkle the plums, in their 50 per cent 'mead nectar', with two tablespoons of sugar and a little powdered cinnamon.
Cover the bowl and let it steep for a day, ideally by bouncing it over potholed Baltic roads.
In the evening, microwave the plums for two and a half minutes then mix immediately with an equal quantity of chilled Lithuanian soured cream.
The hot and cold combination is extremely good. Consume with locally purchased, vanilla essence, sponge fingers.

Wholly unexpectedly, the campsites in Lithuania were outstandingly good. I'd picked up the very short list of them in Druskininkai and now I was on a deeply wooded peninsula on Lake Galve in Trakai National Park, only 20 kilometres from Vilnius where I was heading the next day to speak

221

to the Golden Retriever Breeders' Club of Lithuania. This was the largest campsite I stayed at in the Baltic, room for around 100 motorhomes but also innumerable cottages, cabins and dormitories. A tour bus with Russian licence plates arrived just after I did, but otherwise there was only one other motorhome, with German plates, parked at the distant far end of the bowl-shaped grassy camping sector.

A cold northerly rain had returned in the late-afternoon and as the wind blew thousands of cold piercing needles into my face, Macy raced and rolled with delight in the grass. We wandered to the sandy lake shore and she tore into the water, biting its surface, prancing like a rocking horse. Some dogs are heat seekers and other live to be wet; Macy's on the latter team. Back at the Roadtrek, while I towelled down inside, she preferred to lie outside in the rain and contemplate nature.

That evening I had dinner in the camp's large log-cabin restaurant. I was the only guest and ordered herring with sour cream, sliced onions, hot boiled potatoes, tomato and a dill pickle as my starter followed by two large perch fillets, lightly breaded and fried, with boiled rice, another dill pickle and finely chopped cabbage with vinegar dressing as my main course.

Although I was the only guest eating, waiters were busy preparing food and drink and a DJ was setting up coloured strobe lights. A man in his thirties—beer-bellied, round-faced, receding hair, too tight jeans, Nike shoes—was overseeing the preparations for the evening and drinking beer drawn from a large keg. We'd made eye contact when I'd entered the restaurant and now he was sitting at a table watching a bleached blonde, big-boobed girl in a clinging top and low-slung jeans dance alone to the music as the DJ continued to fiddle with his lights and test the speakers.

The thirty-something man went to the keg, poured himself another beer then filled another half-litre paper cup and brought it over to me, raised his own cup in a toast and we drank to each other. A few minutes later he returned and this time we clinked our paper cups and he said '*Zwei katzen*'. I thought 'Two cats' in German was a pretty weird toast but I repeated it back. He grinned and corrected me, '*Sveikata!*' When he brought a third beer to the table and we toasted again, I asked him to join me and we watched the attractive girl continue to gyrate on the dance floor, seductively lost in her own thoughts.

People started to fill the restaurant, more neatly dressed thirty-somethings. In halting English my friend explained that he was a tour operator. 'Russian. Moscow,' he said gesturing at the almost formal crowd now taking seats at the tables around the room. Over the next beer and '*Sveikata!*' he nodded towards the girl shaking her enormous chest on the dance-floor. 'Mine,' he explained, and I nodded and winked in approval. 'Congratulations,' I replied, riveted by the seemingly endless variety of directions two boobs could take in such an exquisitely short period of time. The dancer had picked up the microphone and now she had it close to her scarlet lips and was singing into it. Well, no. She was licking it. 'My sister,' the tour operator said, nodding

223

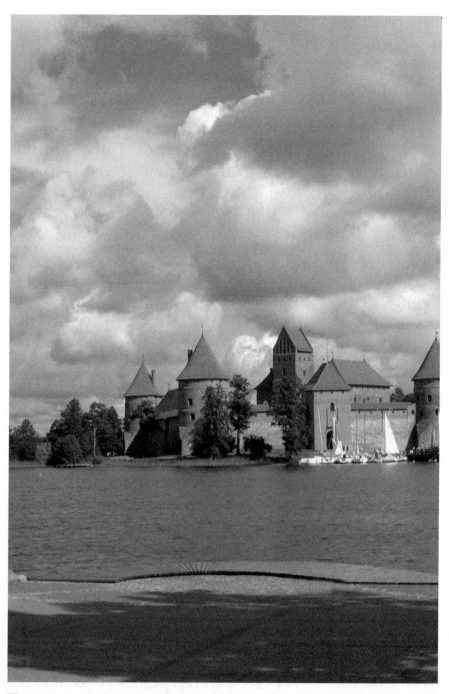

THE FANTASY CASTLE AT TRAKAI, COMPLETED IN 1987

approvingly.

It was a family business. The tour operator managed the logistics and his sister and her boyfriend provided the entertainment. He brought coach loads of singleton Muscovites here each weekend during the summer. This was the last party of the season.

The Muscovites danced in an old-fashioned way. The guys held their partners formally as they danced two-steps and foxtrots. During a break the tour operator's sister came to the table and we were introduced. She was a sociology graduate, had a car and a good job and told me she loved Lithuania because of the dramatic seasons. She had been to Italy and Spain and didn't like the way men there treated her as if she were a visiting prostitute. I was going to point out that her presentation package wasn't exactly kept under wraps but I asked instead how old she was and she told me 24.

She asked me how old I was and I didn't lie.

'Baltic men don't have teeth like yours. How can you have skin like that? Baltic men would never travel alone with a dog. That is wonderful. In Lithuania people your age think of nothing— perhaps what to eat. Golden retriever. That is my favourite breed. May I meet her?'

Was this a come-on? I didn't know what to make of it, but now, at the mention of dogs, two of the Russians, a man and a woman at the table joined in.

'You have golden retriever? From England? Here?'

And so four Muscovites, a Lithuanian and I trooped out to the Roadtrek for a visit with Macy.

225

The cuddles were outrageous and unfortunately I was not included in them—the slobbering Slavic hugs were all reserved for my dog. We trooped back to the restaurant afterwards and while I was talking some more with the Russians, my son Ben telephoned to see how I was.

'What's that music?' he asked listening to the pulsing Slavic rock in the background, then giggled and said, 'Sounds like you're OK. I'll speak to you tomorrow,' laughed again and was gone.

It was absolutely, positively freezing the next morning. I went to the shower house and hot showered for as long as I had litas to put in the coin receptacle. Macy was pissed off that I had gone for so long before her morning walk and of course I was just pissed. And I had to speak at the Golden Retriever Breeders' Club of Lithuania, in Vilnius later in the day.

There was an extraordinary blue morning haze—or maybe it was my bleary eyes—but for whatever reason the mist over the lake at sunrise was inspiring. A hangover soon clears when you walk through damp woods in fresh invigorating air to the water's edge and see ducks gliding silently through the mist, and the flickering light of a night fisherman's campfire glimmering on a peninsula of land so thin that each tree stands out in sharp silhouette.

The meadows by the lake, beyond the woodland, where Macy exercised, were filled with blue chicory, yellow St John's wort and long stemmed plantain. In the lake where she drank were bulrushes and water lilies. Trakai, a 15-minute drive away, on the south side of the lake is a picturesque town built on a peninsula touching three lakes. Its stunning backdrop is a red-brick, turreted and watch-towered Disneyesque castle around 500 metres offshore on an island in Lake Galve.

The castle is, in fact, every bit as historic as Walt Disney. It was first built in the thirteenth century but had fallen into ruins by the eighteenth; the stonework scavenged for use in other buildings. In 1930 the Lithuanian government made an initial effort to preserve what was left, and in 1956 the government started to rebuild the castle. The problem was, no one could agree on what the rebuilt castle should look like. The compromise was this fantasy, of the type of castle King Vytautas might have lived in during the twelfth century when this was the heart of Lithuania. It was completed in 1987.

Simonas had told me there is a vanishingly small sect of Jews in Trakai—the Karaim –who speak, or at least until his generation, spoke their own Turkic language, an audible reminder that Jews had first emigrated here from central Asia in the eighth century. Only a few hundred Karaim survive and their culture will inevitably die with this generation.

*   *   *

I tried to buy groceries in Trakai but the selection in the supermarket was abysmal and I left. The hand-stitched linen tablecloths for sale amongst the ubiquitous amber jewellery in the market stalls on the lakeside were inexpensive, practical and attractive. Seeing me buy a couple, a Japanese tourist did so too.

On the Trakai to Vilnius road, passing through pine woodland, I stopped to buy mushrooms from an old *babushka* sitting by the roadside. I'd passed many more before I stopped for her. These old women, sitting silently by the shoulder of the road, wrapped in thick layers of clothing, were more frequent than road signs.

Her headscarf was pulled so far down over her face I only saw the thin slits of her eyes when she looked up at me. Her vein-burst skin was tight and shiny. She had two plastic boxes, recycled supermarket containers, with mixed mushrooms in them and with hand signals I asked how much she wanted. She showed me 10 fingers, twice, and I gave her 20 litas, a little more than five euros.

'Spaseeba,' she said, breaking the silence. 'Spaseeba.' 'Thank you, thank you,' in Russian.

There aren't many Russians in Lithuania. While they make up one third of the population in Latvia, half the population in Riga alone, they are a small minority here in Lithuania—less than 10 per cent, and almost all in cities.

I thought it might be nice to give her something she'd never seen before, so I returned to the Roadtrek and got an unopened packet of Marks & Spencer Viennese biscuits—part of my strategic reserve. As I returned to give them to her Macy jumped out of the door and, tail raised, joined me. She walked over to the old lady and simply and quietly sat down in front of her, facing her.

My dog can be a calm, still, individual, sometimes irritatingly so. She doesn't wear her emotions visibly. She looked at the old woman and the old woman looked at my dog and then she lifted a thick, puffy hand and stroked Macy's head.

She lifted her other hand and buried her stubby, cracked fingers in the hair on my dog's neck. I sat down, silent too.

'*Kraseevy*,' she said. '*Kraseevy*.' Later that day I learned it simply meant, 'Beautiful. Beautiful.'

With both hands she stroked my dog and all the while Macy just sat still, never revealing what she was thinking. I looked at the old woman's face and tears were rolling down her shiny cheeks like peas. Soon they came from my eyes too.

*   *   *

Arturas Abromavicius and his daughter Dovile had arranged to meet me on the highway near Vilnius to guide me through the town to a hotel north of the city where I was speaking that afternoon. I almost missed them. Lost in thoughts about the mushroom picker, I raced past Arturas's Nissan 4WD parked on the verge of the road, only realising I'd missed him when he caught up with me a kilometre further on. We introduced ourselves and I followed him through Vilnius to the Baltpark Hotel on the main highway heading north-east out of the city towards Ukmergė.

Vilnius is surprisingly and wonderfully hilly and forested. Road signs for Minsk, across the nearby Belarus border, reminded me that I was, by the most recent definition, on the 'edge of Europe'. The gleaming glass and aluminium Saab, Peugeot and Volvo showrooms that lined the highway and the confidently robust, 30-storey skyscrapers on the horizon to the east were not what I had expected to see in the city of my ancestors. I could easily have been on a highway on the outskirts of a successful German city, but for the myriad young hitchhikers with their thumbs out at each traffic light.

The TV tower that sprouted from a far-off hill to my left, surmounted by a revolving restaurant, was more familiar. It is only 15 years since I watched the news and saw Soviet tanks, sanctioned by Mikhail Gorbachev attack crowds at that tower in 1991, killing or injuring hundreds after Vytautas Landsbergis declared Lithuanian independence from the Soviets. Lithuania was the first Soviet republic to break away.

There was a further attack by Soviet forces on a Lithuanian frontier post 20 kilometres away on the highway to Minsk, killing more, but after that the Russians stopped further military action and Lithuania found itself independent. The people I was driving to meet had suddenly and unexpectedly had their futures dramatically changed.

Now—according to French geographers—I was close to the true centre of Europe, which lay less than 20 kilometres to the north. This, they claim, is the geographical centre of the European continent, equidistant from the Atlantic and the Urals, the Arctic and the Mediterranean.

The Baltpark Hotel is yet one more gleaming new building, surrounded by grass and trees, set back from the freshly tarmacked new highway. Macy had a quick roll on the grass, to a backdrop forest of decaying, suburban, Soviet era, grey concrete apartment blocks sprouting amongst the trees of the surrounding hills. Arturas explained to me that the only significance of the use of grey bricks throughout the Baltic States was that silica, from which they are made, is plentiful and cheap in the region.

Arturas Abromavicius is a hydrogeologist, born in the port city of Klaipėda on the Baltic coast. Dovile Abromaviciute is his 'eligible' daughter. I know she's eligible because when I asked her why her last name was different from her father's she explained that her mother's name, Abromaviciene, indicated 'married' while hers indicated 'single'. There were alternative choices for her which also indicated her availability: Abromavicaite and Abromavicyte. More recently, the Lithuanian equivalent of 'Ms' was created, so Dovile and her mother both could choose to be known as Abromavica or Abromavice but few Lithuanian women are choosing these options.

Arturas' father was a sailor and his mother worked in a wood-processing factory. He chose hydrogeology mostly because he didn't like the prospect of working in an office and knew that hydrogeology would always involve fieldwork. As a university student he assumed he would work for a government authority, hopefully in ground water management but in the 1980s he was amongst those of his generation who sensed that independent thought or action was possible.

Gorbachev had opened the door a little, raising the possibility that one could speak one's own mind. That made people like Arturas think that it might be possible to express their own opinions, even to criticise the system. Instead of opting for a government job—the only work that was permitted in Soviet culture—Arturas became an activist, a protester, a campaigner, a green.

In Lithuania, environmentalists were not

considered a big threat to the system and so when young scientists from the Academy of Science started to organise clubs and groups where environmental issues were discussed, there was no opposition from the Communist Party. When these group discussions evolved into meetings, actions and picketing involving thousands of youth, the Party reacted but by then it was too late. People with a political agenda became actively involved and the Green Movement became an independence movement.

With independence it was now possible not just to protest but to 'do', and Arturas set up an environment management business, and considering his evolution from activist to entrepreneur, it's appropriately named *Alternatyva*'. His first contract—with the new Lithuanian government—was to investigate and catalogue fuel, ordinance and chemical ground contamination on former Soviet military bases. Funds for those investigations came from Scandinavian countries, Denmark in particular, that had a vested interest in knowing exactly what might end up in their half of the Baltic Sea. That lead to contacts with Danish and Swedish environment management companies and eventually to their involvement in his business venture.

Arturas got a golden retriever after reading about the breed in the Lithuanian edition of one of the books I'd written. I'd chanced, completely by accident, on Arturas and his daughter Dovile, when I saw an '.lt' address on a golden retriever breeders' website and emailed them.

We choose dogs that look or behave in ways that

232

are compatible with or comforting to our personalities, and Arturas, in a creased, cream linen jacket and a three-day growth of beard sure wasn't a poodle owner. He's a 'doer', setting up his business, the golden retriever club, and a local branch of Lions Club for that matter. As Macy jumped from the Roadtrek, he gave her a warm pummelling and instantly played retrieve with her, throwing a fluorescent ring into the surrounding grassy hills for her to retrieve.

Assembled at the hotel for the afternoon was an elegant selection of golden retriever owners, all of whom were familiar with the breed's medical problems and personality traits. While I talked and answered questions, mostly asked in English, Mace cruised the room, accepting body rubs and softly spoken words. We all had coffee and cakes that Arturas had arranged.

During the talk I'd explained that around 20 years ago a culture shift occurred in London and that most people now clean up after their dogs. I pulled a neatly folded Tesco bag from my back pocket to illustrate that I had my Boy Scout badge in poop-scooping. Everyone in the room pulled out their own plastic bags, a great display of one-upmanship. After the talk, Arturas asked if he could have the bag and he collected all the surplus pastry into it. 'You and Macy can enjoy this,' he explained. He filled another bag with the teabags and bottles of mineral water we hadn't consumed. I liked that. I hate waste.

*   *   *

Vilnius was well preserved during Soviet times, for

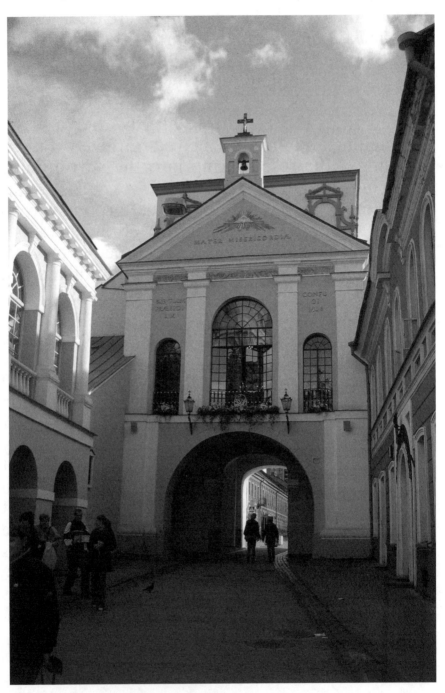

THE GATE OF DAWN, VILNIUS

the sake of Soviet bloc tourism, and is now being transformed to appeal to Western European tourists. The infrastructure changes are obvious—vistas of the city from the surrounding hills have been created and Soviet era buildings removed.

Arturas and Dovile took me for a walk through the old town. It was charming, elegant, sophisticated and beautiful after the grey, bleak ugliness of Kaunas. This is an historic frontier town, the easternmost stronghold of the Catholic church and it is a great Baroque survivor. Its population was historically Polish, Jewish, German, Lithuanian, and Armenian, but most of the population today arrived under Soviet rule.

Arturas parked near the Gate of Dawn, the only surviving city gate, and we visited the hauntingly beautiful, glitteringly opulent, silver-clad Madonna of the Gate. It was off-season but even so there was a queue to enter the narrow staircase that led up to the chamber where the image of the Madonna is housed. It is a small room but the floor was as densely packed with kneeling supplicants whispering prayers and crossing themselves, as a mosque on Friday in a traditional Islamic country. They prayed quietly, passively, individually, undisturbed by the gentle shuffle of our passing feet.

'Of course this was once a great Jewish city, almost half the population,' Arturas mentioned as we walked from the gate through the town hall square, 'but few vestiges of that fact remain.' The surrounding colour-washed, orange, burgundy and blue town houses date from the late 1700s, 100 years after my great-great-great-great-great-great-grandfather 'Itchi' was born somewhere in the streets and alleyways just 50 metres to my right. The Madonna of the Gate chapel was built in 1671 and had been standing for only 19 years when my oldest-known ancestor was born here.

Arturas and Dovile took me to a rustic restaurant, exactly the type of place I'd expect a golden retriever owner to enjoy. I didn't want to compromise our relationship so I held back on questions about life in Lithuania today but I did mention the mushroom picker I had met that morning.

'Pensioners are the losers with the changes that have taken place. The government has left them to care for themselves. Prices rise but many have not enough money to pay even for heat in winter. You know, Lithuania depends on natural gas from Russia. The Russians do not have to invade us to control us. They are more sophisticated now. They are trying to control us by manipulating the economy. The Russian government controls Gazprom and dictates to Gazprom the price of gas to Lithuania.'

While we talked, Arturas took a message on his mobile telephone. It was telling him that the time on his parking-meter was about to expire. He tapped a few keys and extended his parking time. Such is the backwardness of modern Vilnius.

'Vilnius has done well,' he explained. 'There is wealth here but this is an ambitious island in Lithuania. The rest of the country has not yet shared the success of Vilnius. Almost 300,000 Lithuanians have left the country since 1990. I don't see how we can sustain such loss.'

*　　　*　　　*

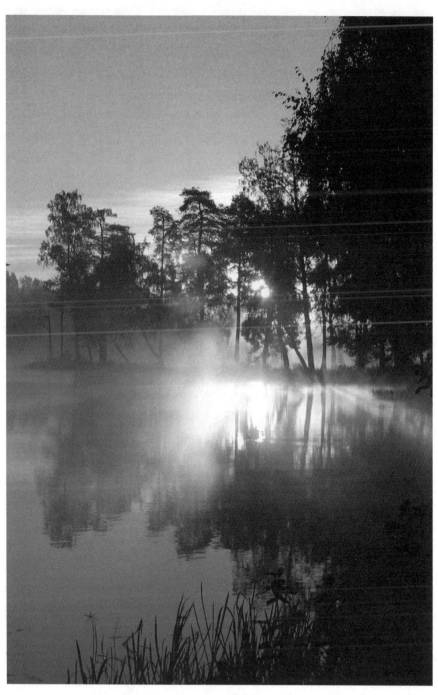

DAWN MIST OVER THE LAKE AT TRAKAI

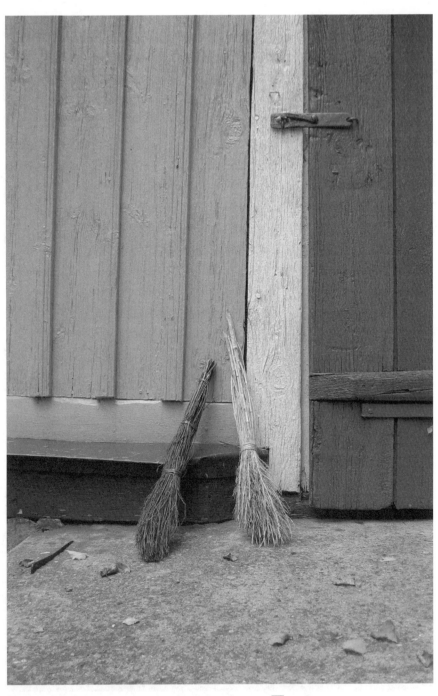

Bessoms on a doorstep near Trakai

A heavy dawn mist drifted off the lake and settled as low fog over the campsite at Trakai. We walked up the hill, above the fog, and Macy pirouetted in the sharp morning light through a field smothered in a glistening crop of cobwebs, the land behind whitewashed into nothingness. It was crisp, fresh and sunny. Last night, after returning to the campsite, Macy had played in the dark for over an hour with a boxer dog, play bowing, leaping, rolling. I don't know where it came from and it disappeared as mysteriously as it arrived but that was the first pleasant dog-to-dog experience Macy had had for a week.

Heading towards Poland I drove through dense blankets of fog on a pristine, new, perfectly banked, black ribbon of highway where even the cuttings that ran through the rolling forest had been carefully turfed with immaculate grass. Horse manure on this newest E road told me that farmers were still using it to get to their fields of potatoes. There were more light-grey cattle here.

The evening before I had met up with a local vet. He had explained to me that there were three decently equipped veterinary clinics in Vilnius, with X-ray and ultrasound facilities, and one in Kaunas. He was hoping to work in Britain. I asked him about cattle and he told me that black and whites were most common but Lithuanian Red cattle still accounted for one-third of the national cattle herd. Light-grey cattle, once common, were now rare, restricted to the south, where I was now travelling.

At 8.30 a.m. people were already digging potatoes from the sandy soil. A farmer was walking one of his cows on a lead along the verge of the highway. The mirror-calm lakes were studded with occasional rowing boats in which solitary men were fishing. There was scant evidence of the Soviet occupation along this road, but the fields were still predominantly fallow. The village of Aukstadvaris was chocolate-box picturesque, its neat wooden buildings sitting amongst the surrounding rolling hills with the placid lakes below, their locations given away by coverings of fog.

The serene smoothness of the new E road ended near where the road bridged the Nemunas River, and I was back on a typical pock-marked road surface. I took a break in the town of Mariampolė, turned right on red lights as is thoughtfully permitted in Lithuania, visited the church and raptly listened to its exquisite women's choir. I shopped in the local Maxima supermarket—as busy as the church—where I bought *challah* bread, macaroons, herring, soured cream and a one-kilogram live carp that I chose from a glass and stainless steel tank in the delicatessen section, and had cleaned and gutted.

I was only a few miles from what is now the border between Lithuania and Poland, although across that border, most people in the region of Poland I was soon to visit spoke Lithuanian. Virtually everywhere I have travelled in Europe there had been border changes in the twentieth century—Germany and Denmark, Finland and Russia, Estonia and Russia, Estonia and Latvia— but now I was in the nerve centre of shifting borders. Lithuania and Latvia; Lithuania and Belarus; Lithuania and Poland; Lithuania and Germany; and after Russia annexed German East

Prussia, Lithuania and Russia, all had been redefined, most in my lifetime. I took the lesser-travelled road towards the town of Sejny in Poland, close to where Lithuania, Poland and Belarus all now meet in dense woodland, at least for the time being.

Just as borders have changed, so too have the people who inhabited this benighted land. Languages have flourished and been extinguished. In Lithuania in my lifetime first Yiddish was expunged, then German and then Polish. Now Russian is being snuffed out and replaced with English. Visit Lithuania and you attend a master class in the rewriting of history. The only place I saw an active mention of Jews was Grūto Parkas.

At that sculpture park, the communist villains are described according to their nationality, Polish, Russian, German, Latvian and for some, 'Nationality—Jewish'. Invariably, they have Lithuanian-ending names like Greifenbergeris or Carnas but they're not 'Nationality—Lithuanian'. To the modern historians of Grūto Parkas there were no Lithuanian communists, only alien, Jewish ones with Lithuanian names.

Travel through this part of Europe and it is transparent there's no such thing as history. The fantasies, the aspirations and ideals, the fears and prejudices, the bigotry and embarrassments of the dominant nationality in a region are what masquerade as history. At Grūto Parkas, the Lithuanian Jews who joined the Communist Party have had their nationality erased. In the Grūto Parkas interpretation of history, their religion has replaced their nationality. You still cannot be both Lithuanian and Jewish.

241

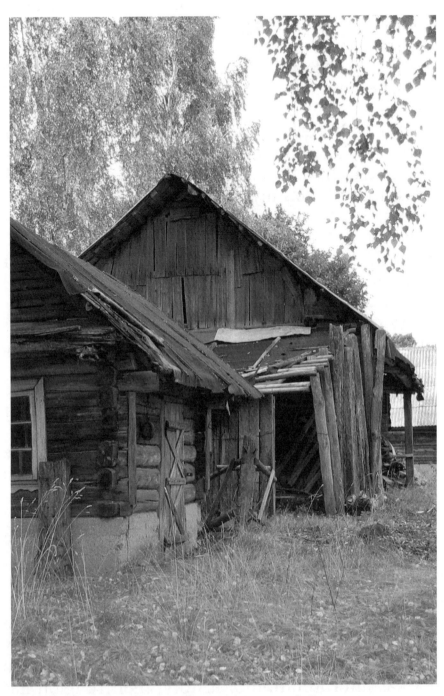

Traditional farm buildings at Margionys

Ironically, both Catholic and Jewish Lithuanians shared similar aspirations. Neither felt they had a nation to which they could attach their strong sense of identity. Both fantasised about idealised, homogeneous nations, countries that would be wholly Lithuanian or wholly Jewish. To Lithuanian nationalists it was, and I suspect still is, incomprehensible to contemplate a Jewish community within their nation that has its allegiance to the Lithuanian state.

Nineteenth and early twentieth-century Jewish romantics and idealists argued that the only way to avoid anti-Semitism in Europe was for Jews to have their own safe and independent homeland, in Israel. Zionists believed that anti-Semitism itself would wither and die when Jews at last had a Jewish state.

Theodor Herzl wrote that 'A wondrous breed of Jews will spring up from the earth. We shall live at last as free men on our own soil, and in our homes peacefully die.' In his negotiations in Constantinople with the Ottoman Sultan, the ruler of Palestine, he explained that the Jews likely to emigrate would be 'sober, industrious and loyal . . . bound to the Muslims by racial kinship and religious affinity.' Such was the uplifting optimism of early Zionism. Would Herzl recognise Israel today?

I am proud that the culture I was raised in is one that emphasised—idealised—asking questions, questioning answers, gaining knowledge, learning more, all enveloped in the warm cloak of family. The shivering, shock of reality is that my culture, my Jewish European heritage, is really no more intellectually rigorous than any other. All of us are

243

susceptible to the biological reality of tribalism.

Only the civilising consequences of culture can possibly overcome our latent nationalism. The insoluble intolerance of so many Muslims and Jews to each other today, their hostility to the very presence of 'others' living amongst them exists because in the twentieth century dormant ethnicity was unleashed in both populations.

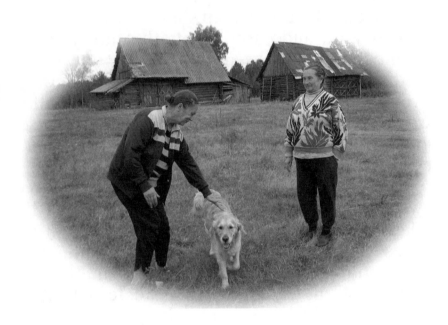

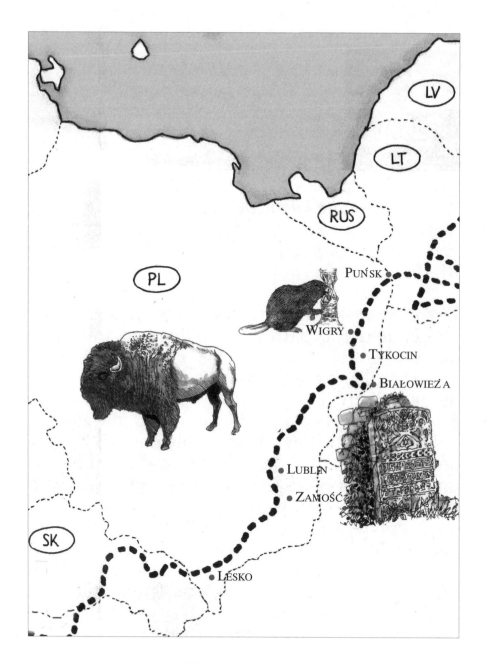

CHAPTER SEVEN

POLAND

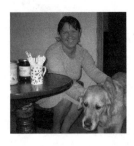

POLAND

People per square kilometre	*123*
Dogs per square kilometre	*19*
Reconstructed fake animal species	*2*
Wolves	*750*

Despite the heavy-duty document checks at the border and the patrolling soldiers in full battle fatigues, I was glad to be in Poland. It seemed more familiar to me, a country I recognised if only because there were so many people with Polish origins in the place where I was raised in Canada.

Here I was in what is probably one of the most unvisited, remote, and, in a captivating way, unspoilt corners of Europe. Stork nests sat atop purpose-built platforms on utility poles. Rolling open countryside interspersed with pine forests and small lakes lay in all directions as I travelled the rutted road to the market town of Sejny, where the elegant 'multicultural centre'—once the main synagogue, was used as a fire station by the Germans in World War Two.

I took narrow back roads to Puńsk where Mass—performed in Lithuanian—had just finished. The interior of the neo-Gothic church was decorated with dozens of wild herb and flower garlands suspended in giant hoops from the rafters. This corner of Poland remains ethnically mixed: Poles, Lithuanians, Russians, Belarusians and Ukrainians all live here. While walking Macy I saw a sign saying '*Miód—Medus*' and followed it to a new breeze-block house where grass had yet to be laid in the garden. Jolanta answered the door and when I said '*Miód?*' she replied, '*Deutsch?*' and beckoned me in.

Macy and I were escorted to a sitting-room where Jolanta had set four jars of honey and some tasting spoons on a coffee table. With Jolanta's permission Macy wandered out of the room, following the rich aroma of meat stew simmering in the kitchen. One of the flowing honeys had an almost minty sweetness to it but I opted for a jar of bright, lemon-curd yellow, set honey. Macy returned to the tasting room, licking her lips, accompanied by Jolanta's smiling mother who bubbled enthusiastically to Jolanta, who in turn explained to me that Macy was the best-looking stray dog to ever wander in to her kitchen.

*　　　*　　　*

This north-west corner of Poland was once the Russian province of Suwalki, 'Suwalki Guberniya' and, although there were as many cats and dogs wandering these back roads as there were across the border in Lithuania, farming looked considerably different here. There were many more fenced fields and, for the first time since Finland, I saw a line of cattle untethered, walking free—probably to the milking shed. Tethered cows were still in the majority however, and many of them had churns sitting ready next to them out in

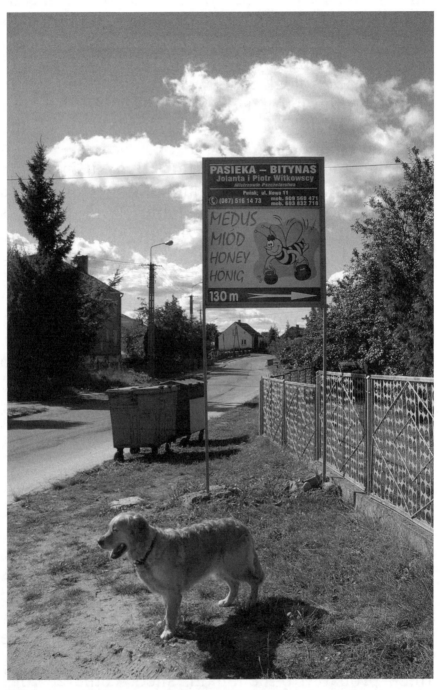

WHILE WALKING MACY I SAW A SIGN SAYING
'*MIÓD—MEDUS*'

the fields.

One spectacular-looking heifer had a mushroom-grey body and a creamy white head. She was stunning. Fields were smaller than in Lithuania and most open land was not fallow as in all the Baltic states but under cultivation—mostly harvested with some winter crops already seeded, just turning green. White plastic-covered spools of straw were stacked neatly on many farms. As is the case everywhere that cattle are kept, bathtubs were used as water troughs and dotted the fields. In open woods by a marsh in Wigierski National Park I set up camp early and wondered where mosquitoes went when the temperature suddenly dropped, as it did that night.

North of the town of Suwalki, so far off the beaten path that you have to walk on a dirt track for an hour to get there, is Wodziłiki, a rustic collection of homes and farm buildings in a wooden valley inhabited by Old Believers, whose culture I'd first encountered in Estonia. The following morning, on another cloudless day, I headed back north-west towards the Lithuanian border and Wodziłiki.

A raptor flew in front of the Roadtrek from the cover of the surrounding pine trees, looked straight into my eyes then rocketed up and away. On these back roads there were many new houses, often with varying geometric motifs painted on them and at Jeleniewo there was a neo-Gothic wooden Catholic church built so recently that the wood had only just started weathering. Inside, the smell of fresh-cut lumber was intoxicating. Morning light cascaded through the east-facing stained glass windows, showering the interior in wonderful, warm autumn colours. I got out my phrase book and said 'Hello' to the workmen in Polish. They replied that no, they took their coffee black.

It took some trial and error before I found a track where I could park. Barry, my Sat Nav buddy, who didn't know the Baltic states at all, knew Poland but not intimately. He was fine as long as I stuck to main roads. When we did manage to pull over, Macy and I hiked north along a dirt track through flowering meadow and pine forest following road signs towards Wodziłki.

The path passed close to an ancient thatched barn, the walls made from large, rough hewn granite rocks each over 60 centimetres in diameter. As we neared the far end of the barn a ferocious looking 40-kilogram brute of a farm dog emerged and, slobbering saliva and screaming obscenities, launched himself into the air towards us, coming to an abrupt mid-air stop when he reached the end of his thick rope tether. We were as safe as his rope was strong.

Behind him, by a large dog house adjacent to another rustic farm building, another guard dog lunged forward until restrained by his chain tether, then turned and climbed the granite wall as high as he could, and bounced off it in another lunge towards us. He repeated the manoeuvre again and again stereotypically. At the end of the field, when I turned and looked back, he was still bouncing off the wall.

*   *   *

The Slavs were converted to Christianity by

Byzantine missionaries—initially by the brothers Methodius and Cyril who created the modern Russian alphabet, 'Cyrillic', and encouraged the use of vernacular languages in church liturgy. Each region of the Orthodox Church developed its own individuality.

The Old Believers are a sect that opposed the liturgical reforms, that were adopted by the Russian Orthodox church in the seventeenth century such as wearing Greek ecclesiastical dress and using three fingers instead of two when making the sign of the cross.

To escape religious persecution, Old Believers moved as far as possible from the eyes of the Russian Orthodox church, to the fringe of the Russian empire: Suwalki Guberniya. They survived in large numbers until World War Two when the area came under German occupation. The men's long beards and the way they dressed meant that they were mistaken by the Germans for Jews. Most Polish Old Believers fled to Lithuania and only a few returned after the war. I was told that their place of worship, their original 'molenna' in Wodziłiki, survived and that they lived, not unlike Old Order Mennonites in Ontario, in rural houses devoid of modern amenities such as indoor plumbing.

Hovering red dragonflies followed Macy like a squadron of miniature helicopters as she trotted through the ditches and fields along the road. For entertainment she pounced on grasshoppers, a new game for her, and once more found a black slimy bog to wallow in. At a fork in the road the sign to the village had fallen but was propped up and pointed to the right. I followed that track for half an hour before emerging from dense pine woodland to realise that there were no fresh footprints on the track and that the sign had been intentionally moved, probably to keep tourists like me away. I didn't mind because I was by a potato field and there were no potato pickers about.

In Denmark I'd bought new potatoes from a roadside stand. In Finland I found dark purple potatoes in a local supermarket but ever since arriving in Estonia and seeing such a cottage industry of potato growing, I wanted to find out exactly what type of potatoes families were harvesting from their family plots. I had stopped by a family of pickers in Lithuania but the language barrier was so overwhelming I got nowhere. The uprooted sign at the road junction gave me a chance to investigate the 15 brown burlap and white woven plastic bags filled with potatoes, and perhaps acquire some.

Poland is the world's second largest producer of potatoes but this is a relatively recent phenomenon. For years the peasants actually resisted demands by their rulers to grow potatoes. Their diet was black, brown and grey bread made from rye, oats and barley. Bread was sacred. It was the Communion. It was Christ's body. These ugly, tuberous root vegetables on the other hand had no sanctity and were scarcely innocent. What was uniquely frightening to peasants was that not only did a plant grow from seed, but it also grew mysteriously—devilishly—from a grotesque tuber.

According to local superstition, potatoes caused women to menstruate or lactate and men to produce sperm. From the West, the Prussian King Frederick the Great ordered potatoes to be grown

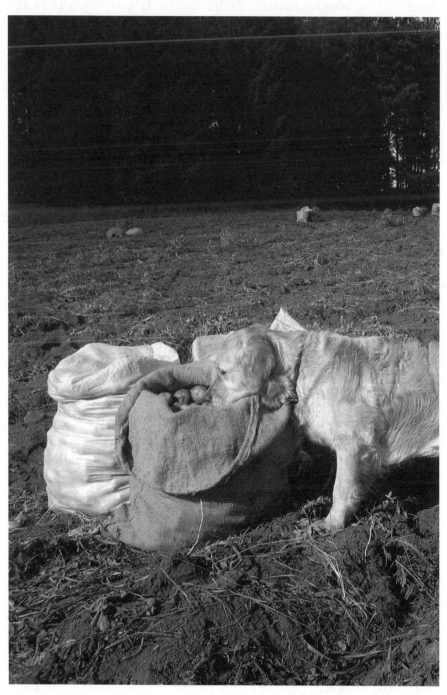

Macy checks out potatoes at Wodziłiki

as a safeguard against famine in the 1770s but the peasants refused. The town of Kolberg sent him a message, 'The things have neither smell nor taste, not even the dogs will eat them, so what use are they to us?'

From the East, the Orthodox church was opposed to growing potatoes and Catherine the Great of Russia had to overrule the Orthodox fundamentalists and instruct her peasants to grow potatoes. They refused. It was not until 1850, when Tsar Nicholas I compelled the peasants by decree to grow potatoes that local Christian farmers joined their Jewish neighbours, who had not had religious objections either to growing or to eating these alien roots. Old Believers continued to reject potatoes, calling them 'Devil's apples' or 'forbidden fruit'.

Phytophthora infestans, the fungal potato blight that lead to the great famine in Ireland in 1848, reached Poland too, turning stems and tubers into a putrid mess, and making entire fields scorched and black in a week. But as in Ireland, Polish potato breeders found resistant stock, used the seed pods to create healthier stock and by the turn of the twentieth century even Old Believers were growing them. They ate potatoes roasted on embers, seasoned with salt. The better-off sliced potatoes, powdered them in flour and fried them in butter. Jewish mothers, with a longer tradition of cooking with potatoes, fried, boiled or baked them in their own unique but simple ways.

POTATO KNEIDLACH
Grate peeled potatoes and squeeze out excess moisture.

Beat in eggs, finely chopped onion, salt and matzo flour.
Form dumplings and cook in boiling water.

POTATO LATKES
Grate peeled potatoes and squeeze out excess moisture.
Beat in eggs and salt.
Form pancakes and fry in vegetable oil until crispy brown on both sides.

POTATO KUGEL
Grate peeled potatoes and squeeze out excess moisture.
Beat in egg yolks, finely chopped onion, salt and crumbled matzo.
Beat in egg whites, mix thoroughly, press into a greased pie dish and bake in the oven until the surface is crisp.

Potatoes arrived in Spain in 1570 from South America where they had been farmed in the Andes for perhaps 7000 years. They were named 'cartoufle' by a Frenchman, Olivier de Serres, who simply corrupted the Italian word for truffle, 'tartufi', and this is the source of their Polish name, 'kartoffel', and also their name in languages as diverse as Danish, Russian and German. Later, to improve the root's image, Burgundian entrepreneurial growers nicknamed the potato the 'pomme de terre'.

The obvious advantage of the potato is its hardiness. The starchy tubers can feed the plant and keep it alive during all but the most severe frosts and even during droughts over seven months

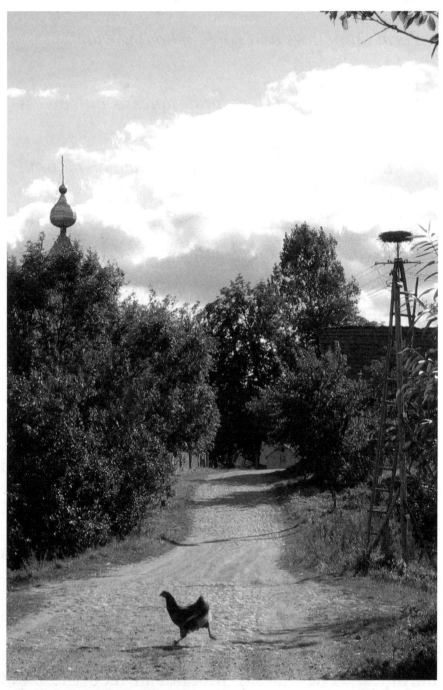

WODZIŁIKI: THE ONION DOME OF THE MOLENNA
ROSE ABOVE THE TREES

long. They grow in the poorest soils and need little attention once they are planted. Best of all, from the military strategist's perspective, they can't be as easily destroyed as wheat, barley, rye or any other cereal crop if the enemy uses a scorched-earth policy.

*   *   *

The potatoes collected and bagged in this field were unexceptional looking. They had thin brown skins and numerous eyes. Even so, they were fresh and they were local. Using the trusty doggy bag I always keep in my back pocket, I selected a dozen and nestled a five złłoty coin as payment on to the most prominent and the flattest potato in one of the burlap sacks.

Backtracking to the fork in the road I reached Wodziłiki. The onion dome of the *molenna* rose above the trees on one side of the path and a stork's nest on a platform atop a utility pole on the other. Chickens clucked and scurried across in front of me. The wooden *molenna* was immaculate, fully restored with a new concrete base and roofed in lead. What a pity. I was hoping for something more rustic.

The farm buildings along the path and in the dells on either side were thatch-roofed with yards filled with typical farm junk: ancient tractors, handmade pitchforks and rakes made from straight, thin tree saplings, white plastic buckets and old bits of rusting metalwork or lumber. And dogs. Each barnyard had a chained dog and all of them did their job with dedication. It would have been idyllic if only the ambience had not been polluted by so much angry barking.

* * *

The beaver is the symbol of Wigry National Park and I returned there to spend the rest of the day camping at an 'agrotourism' farm where the most Hollywood-gorgeous young woman, dark-haired, Caribbean-blue eyed, and with a pristine figure in a light cotton, form-hugging print dress and bare feet sashayed me to where I could park. I'd swap my dog for her.

I found it difficult to leave that campsite but Macy implored me to walk her and we departed for an afternoon hike through the fields and villages around the top of the lake. We passed men fishing from docks amongst the reeds on the shore and dogs in yards that went demented trying to attack Macy, who I'm pleased to say took their aggression with aplomb. She simply sailed on by, tail high.

A track went past old farm buildings and wooden homes interspersed with apple orchards. It climbed up into the rolling hills and continued through woodland and field, before descending once more to the reed-lined shore and more isolated farm buildings. Here too there was a profusion of apple trees all heavy with tasty red fruit. Further south the track circled round a marshy extension of the lake. The land was flat and drainage channels had been dug in the harvested fields and in one of those drainage channels was a dam—a beaver dam.

Beaver used to thrive in this part of Europe. One folk memory of their local presence is found in the beaver-skin hats still worn today by the mystic Chassidic Jews in New York, Antwerp or Jerusalem who trace their ancestry to this region. In Canada I have seen beaver homes and superbly engineered beaver dams but I have never, in my life, seen a beaver in the wild. This was the titchiest of dams, only a metre wide, made more from forest debris than from actively chewed-off branches, but there was a beaver somewhere around here and I decided to stay until I saw it.

Beaver once inhabited the whole of Europe. In London, Beverley Brook on the south bank of the Thames is named for them, a reminder that beaver once populated what is now the heart of the London. Here in Poland there are similar place-name reminders: nearby Biebrza, Bobrek, Bobrka in Carpathia, where I was heading. Because beavers have scaly tails, medieval Polish monks who wouldn't eat meat classified them as fish so they could eat them. Discharge from their scent glands, 'castoreum' was medicinal magic, treating female hysteria, fainting, headaches, even helping women deliver their babies. If you have ever smelled their scent gland discharge—I have in zoo beavers—it is easy to understand how castoreum works. You'll do anything to get away from the odour.

In medieval Poland, beaver hunting was reserved for the nobility. A duke's 'beaver hunter' was responsible for ensuring that beavers had the best environments to breed in while the 'beaver master' was in charge of the hunters and the hunt. There's a curious analogy today. The protection of the beaver that made the dam I was now watching is the responsibility, not of a government ministry

259

but of the Polish Hunting Association. The medieval nobles' monopoly on hunting beavers eventually ended and over the following centuries their numbers declined until by the end of the nineteenth century the Polish beaver was virtually extinct. The twentieth century brought protection and at the onset of World War Two there were around 400 survivors but by the end of the war there were not much more than 100, mostly in this region.

In the mid-1970s environmental scientists and the Polish Hunting Association banded together to create a plan to improve local habitats and encourage the repopulation of the country with beavers, especially in the north-eastern region I was in. They developed methods for catching, transporting and settling beaver in regions where water quality was good and there was ample food for survival. Imports of Russian beavers augmented the small numbers available in Poland, and widened the genetic pool.

In less than 30 years beavers virtually saturated all habitable territories, so much so that in some regions, where their compulsive need to build dams has resulted in local flooding, they are now captured and transferred to other regions of Poland not yet inhabited by local beaver populations. Now there are at least 18,000 and rising, over 10,000 of which are in this region of the country alone. The re-emergence of the beaver is one of the untold natural history successes of Polish environmentalists.

Better still, Polish beavers, just like the Poles themselves are now working abroad. A surplus that cannot find work building dams in Poland are working in Germany, Austria, the Netherlands and Slovakia, as breeding stock for the re-beavering of those countries. An organisation in Scotland is hoping for permission to use Polish beavers in a repopulation plan for that part of the UK.

I sat on beaver watch for a long time. Macy went to sleep. Nothing. Not even the slightest crunch from the adjacent woods. I got bored. I counted crows. I watched magpies. I snoozed. Finally I upped and meandered back to the farm where I made dinner and dallied around, doing vehicle housekeeping I'd been meaning to attend to.

POTATOES, APPLES AND BACON
Wash, quarter and boil freshly dug small new potatoes. No need to skin them.
Peel and cut into chunks the size of the potato quarters an almost equal amount of freshly picked red apples.
After the potatoes have boiled for 10 minutes add the apples and cook until they are soft but have not lost their shape. Remove and drain.
Dice fatty Lithuanian bacon and fry until crisp.
Remove from heat, add the potatoes and apples to the crispy bacon and dripping, swirl around and pour on to a plate and offer a small tasting to your dog.
Sit outside a Canadian motorhome on a Polish farm, eat and dream that the farmer's daughter will come to investigate what smells so good.

It was a cold night. Smoke snaked from the chimneys of houses by the lake as we wandered off along a different track for the ritual morning exercise. Mace found an abandoned red-granite root cellar, a sort of stone igloo covered with a mound of soil and turf, its open iron door firmly embedded in the surrounding vegetation. She sniffed intently at the entrance but refused to enter the black void.

Rustic wooden houses, all with heavily laden apple trees in their gardens, lined both sides of the dirt lane and around 100 metres beyond the last inhabited home we chanced upon an abandoned one. There had been no vandalism. The doors were padlocked and the windows were intact. The grasses, shrubs and weeds growing around the home gave me the impression it had been empty for several years but, curiously, there was no fruit on the apple trees. Every single apple had been harvested.

On the overgrown lawn of the home, were 12 unpainted beehives surrounded by knee-high grass, Georgian doll's-house rectangular, just like those near Druskininkai in Lithuania, less than 50 kilometres away as the stork flies. While I inspected the beehives, all of which I would have bought immediately if they were for sale, Macy found a stick in the long grass and tried to lift it but she couldn't. She did sharp backward yanks, as dogs do, until I went to help her and discovered she had found an old handmade rake. It was obviously abandoned and I wanted it, so I pulled it from its web of grass and, standing it upright beside my body so it wasn't totally obvious that I was stealing it, I walked rigid back to the campsite, opened the back of the vehicle and put the rake in. I'd have to share my bed with it for the rest of the trip.

A local radio station was broadcasting Slavic language Eurovision contenders either in Russian or Belarusian but certainly not in Polish as I headed towards Suwalki and on to Augustów. The main road in this region of the country, the E67 to Białystok, was so deeply grooved from the HGVs that rumble along it that I had to swerve hard to get out of the ruts; it was like getting the tyres off tramlines.

South of Augustów, not far off the main road was another Old Believers' church at Gabowe Grady but once more, not a single person stirred anywhere. Macy found an old wooden Orthodox cross in the cemetery and started dragging it towards me and before anyone noticed the desecration I thought it best to leave. Now that I was off the E67, however, I decided to follow a straight and narrow country road south over arable flatland interspersed with woods.

A fox played chicken with me as I drove through one patch of woodland and it occurred to me that there was little road kill here, especially compared to Sweden and Finland. The road unexpectedly turned west over flat marshy land and crossed the Augustus Canal, where at the lock there was a large carved beaver. I backtracked and after several dead ends at farms, one of which had its own small wooden church no larger than a kitchen, I found a route across a narrow neck of marshy, boggy Biebrański National Park and continued on back roads to Tykocin where, allegedly, there are more nesting stork pairs than anywhere else in Poland.

This is the Podlasie region of eastern Poland. Max Białystok, the Zero Mostel character in *The Producers*, is named after the large, unattractive industrial city to the east of Tykocin. In Tykocin itself, if you believe the Polish tourist office website, there were 23 pairs of storks nesting on roofs, pylons and trees this year and I wanted to see some of them.

I arrived over a cobbled road from the north, over the Narew River, sharing the drive into the town with two horse-drawn hayloads. The pretty rectangular town square is bordered by individual, white painted, wooden houses, too low for a self-respecting stork to nest on. The nearby parish church was taller but devoid of stork nests. I drove off, looking for where they lived.

There are over 40,000 storks in Poland, more than anywhere else in Europe. The tourist board website proudly proclaims that in Europe 'every fourth stork is Polish!' although geographically much smaller Latvia and Lithuania provide a summer home for over 20,000 more of these elegant birds. Most 'Polish storks' live here in the north-east and have done so for centuries. My regional ancestors would have been familiar with their nests, their calls and their mating displays.

A white stork is tall, around a metre long, but weighs not much more than a very large chicken, anything from 2.5 to 4.5 kilograms. Storks adapted well to the human agricultural environment. Our farming methods increased their food supply of rodents, insects and frogs. Pastures, meadows and fish ponds were, and—in rustic areas such as this where farming remains basic—still are like supermarkets to them, like ready meals.

Both stork parents share parental duties and long ago peasants observed and admired the way that the male arrived first and built or repaired the nest then awaited the arrival of the female whom he courted with a head shaking, crouching dance, cementing the bond with an up-down display. Banding studies revealed that storks remain monogamous as long as the partner survives and can successfully breed for over 30 years.

Storks came to be associated with good luck and, of course, with fertility. Storks bring babies. While they used to nest in tall trees and on roof-tops, as I had seen in Lithuania, almost 40 per cent of Polish storks nest on utility poles—usually electricity poles. The consequences include electrocution from touching cables and nest fires caused by short circuits. Environmental organisations build platforms on utility poles to keep storks and their young away from danger and to insure that the electricity supply is not interrupted. I passed several of these platforms but saw no storks nesting on them.

* * *

While driving the cobbled streets, I saw in front of a large, red-tiled baroque building, a parked blue *Policja Volkswagen* van with four jackbooted armed cops leaning against it, smoking fags. By the entrance to the building itself stood an athletic-looking, crop-haired, 25 to 30-year-old man in wraparound shades. He wore jeans and a blue Oxford shirt. You can identify an incognito security guy from 50 paces so I parked and went to ask what was happening.

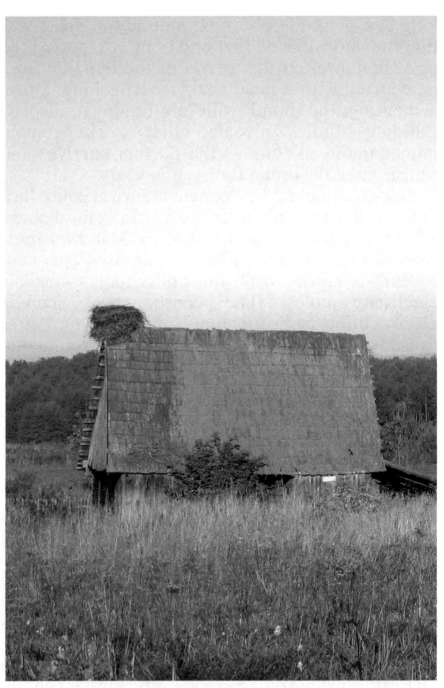

A STORK NEST ON A FARM BUILDING IN TYKOCIN

He explained that he was with a Holocaust tour from Israel, and that the group was inside what was once a synagogue, built in 1642—now a museum—listening to a lecture. The Polish cops were added security from Białystok, laid on because the tourists were Israelis, and when they saw me talking to the Israeli they trooped over and gestured that they would appreciate having their photo taken with the security guy, which I did.

This region of Poland was once heavily populated with Jewish families. I learned that in 1939, over half the population of Tykocin alone was Jewish. Most Polish synagogues, like most Polish churches, were wooden and all of these were destroyed by the Germans but some brick and stone synagogues survived and this one, although heavily damaged, was restored in the 1970s.

It was exceptionally and unexpectedly beautiful inside, with mutely coloured frescoes on the walls making borders to illustrated Hebrew inscriptions—prayers from the Old Testament—which the Israelis could read and understand and I could not. The focus of the room was the central raised *'bimah'*, the place of honour from which prayers are chanted, a large, pillared and arched baroque piece of architecture the arches of which soared to the ceiling and radiated out to join with arches from the walls. It too was painted in predominantly ochre and dirty sky-blue motifs and inscriptions. A dozen heavy brass candelabras hung suspended from the ceiling around the *bimah*, on which a short-sleeved, balding, tawny-haired man was standing speaking with muted emotion. The tourists sat motionless, intent.

The reason I can trace my mother's family, the Breslins, for 10 generations back to Vilnius in 1690 is because they were rabbis by profession. As teachers in a culture that prized piety and learning over wealth and ostentation, their birth and death dates were recorded. Itchi, born in 1690, Reuven, 1710, Chaim, 1753, Yehudah, 1773, another Reuven 1801, another Yehudah, the last of the rabbinical line and the first generation to emigrate to North America, and born in 1835, then my grandfather Chaim, 1876, followed by my mother Aileen, the youngest of 10, born in 1914, me in 1944 and my son Ben in 1973.

That a synagogue as grand as this was built in 1642, spoke of the confidence and the position of the local Jewish community at that time. I know little of where or in what type of synagogues the Breslin rabbis preached. I do know that religion permeated their existence, that it was at the emotional core of life, that it is what created the character and atmosphere of each morning and evening, each weekly Sabbath, each yearly sequence of holy days. Religion dictated every aspect of life, birth, food, puberty, marriage, sex, personal hygiene. Their lives followed a precise list of regulations and rules.

I know that in the 1700s they moved east, to Talacyn, just north of Minsk in what is now Belarus. I have a photo of my great-great-grandfather, born in Talacyn in 1801, died in Talacyn in 1899 and of his son, my great-grandfather born in Talacyn in 1835, died in Toronto only seven years after his father, in 1906. Both show small-featured, white whiskered old men. I've never been able to discern anything about them from their photos but standing in the synagogue in Tykocin and knowing the strong humanist tradition within the Breslin family, I wondered when they first questioned the immutability of their beliefs.

I wondered too about the congregation of Israelis on their Holocaust tour. I hadn't heard that term until Simonas in Kaunas asked me whether I'd like to go on one. I found the idea repellent but now I was observing the reality of their experience and I couldn't help but be moved. Looking at their faces, it was apparent that these people's ancestors came from this part of Europe, as mine did. They were probably listening to a recitation of events that defy understanding, where morality and ethics were so monstrously warped that gratuitous cruelty, merciless brutality, unbearable sadism and mechanical murder were rewarded while compassion, decency, charity, concern, pity, altruism, care, mercy—the qualities shown by the farmers who hid Simonas's grandmother and mother—were punished. It is so awesomely horrific, so mind-numbingly frightening that we are capable of such behaviour, that to avoid confronting that fact, to circumvent the moral vertigo that must come from any reasoned analysis of it, I've found it easier to not think about it. Now I was forced to.

*　　　*　　　*

On a country lane by the Narew River, heading east out of Tykocin towards Białystok, I did see a nesting stork, not yet departed on its flight path over Lebanon and Israel to the base of Africa. It

269

was standing on its nest on a pylon platform, its legs, long and red, its bill straight, red and pointed, its head white. A short distance away was another empty nest, on the edge of a roof. Both nests were massive, certainly wider than I am tall, almost as deep again and constructed of branches and sticks. In the empty one there appeared to be rags or newspaper on one side of it. Both looked relatively new. Mission accomplished.

I drove slowly on the highway back to Białystok, the putrid potential of human behaviour still on my mind. I felt morose. On the way I passed a lean, wrinkled, grey-haired man shovelling the flattened remains of his black-and-white dog off the road while his wife stood watching by the roadside, her crossed arms tightly clenching her sides.

*   *   *

The Białystok region of Poland is home to hundreds of thousands of Belarusians. Advertising billboards are written in Cyrillic as well as Latin script and there is a local Belarusian radio station. Belarus itself owes its existence to Germany. Variously called White Russia, White Ruthenia and Byelorussia, it was a country that didn't exist until Marshal von Hindenburg recognised Byelorussian as an official language in 1916, in what proved to be a successful attempt to wrest the region from under the Russian bear.

The current Republic of Belarus came into existence in 1992 but no motorhome insurer would sell me insurance to take my vehicle there. Cars passing on the highway frequently had Belarus licence plates. I had planned to drive east from Białystok to near the Belarus border and visit one of the villages where there are old wooden Tatar mosques but, not wanting to pass on the opportunity to visit Białowieża in good weather, I travelled directly there, 100 kilometres away.

Białystok had the usual mix of high-rise Soviet era housing which was now painted in flamboyant primary colours, and also new, post-Soviet construction. I saw four brand-new churches on the ring road around the north of the city. Older onion-domed Eastern Orthodox churches were almost as frequent here as Catholic churches. South of Białystok the roadside religious shrines, common everywhere I had travelled in Poland, had Polish flags attached to them and I wondered whether this symbolic equating of nationalism with Catholicism was directed at the minority Orthodox Belarusian community, a not too subtle re-emergence of antipathy towards 'others'. Under Communism, the Catholic church was closely involved in the pro-democracy movement. Is that religious nationalism now spilling over into hostility to minorities and 'outsiders'?

The villages I drove through each had new pink-and-grey pavement stones, reminiscent of the red-and-white national colours. The best-paved roads always lead from the town centre to the local cemetery. The old rectangular wooden houses along the roads were set close together, their narrow sides abutting the road, with their long sides extending deeply back into long, thin lots.

*   *   *

271

'Careful!' Mitek cautioned. I stopped in my tracks, looked around and saw nothing but the invigorating beauty of the surrounding forest. Mitek's eyes motioned down, towards the ground. A step ahead of me on the track I was walking on was a two-centimetre long froglet in green-and-brown army fatigues.

'It is a tree frog. They are common here.'

It was the following day. For Mitek, my personal guide in the closely controlled 'strict reserve' of Białowieski National Park, the forest was like a palliative. As we entered its quiet darkness, the forest revived me too. It was invigorating and animating. It was addictive.

Białowieża is the last large, natural, lowland forest in Europe. It extends over 1260 square kilometres, most of which is on the Belarus side of the border. Here in Poland a large part of the forest is a national park. Most of that park is open to tourists but around 40 per cent is the so-called 'strict reserve', open only to visitors accompanied by a licensed local guide.

The forest survives not just because of its remote location on the fault line between Orthodox and Latin Europe, but because for centuries it was a private hunting ground for a succession of kings and rulers from both sides of Europe's historic divide. As flat as the land may seem—on average only 150 metres above sea level—this is also the hydrological divide between the Baltic Sea to the north-west and the Black Sea to the south-east. There are no lakes in the Białowieża Forest because this is the crown of the Great European Plain.

Considering its uniqueness, not many visitors

come here—fewer than 100,000 annually—but it is only relatively recently that visitors were permitted to come at all. Later in the day Mitek explained that during the Soviet era, when the park was first opened to foreign visitors, guides were instructed to recommend certain restaurants where the tables were bugged so that state security could eavesdrop on naturalists' conversations.

The approach through dense woodlands to Białowieża village was a good taster of what was to come. The road through the village was lined with single storey, red-shingled, occasionally thatched, colour-washed farmhouses most of which had 'zimmer frei' signs on their neat front lawns. Honey was for sale. At the end of the road was a new Best Western hotel, attractively designed as a rustic wooden hunting lodge and beside it was the park's simple tourist office where a fat, wire-haired dachshund ambled over for a tickle while I arranged for a half-day tour of the strict reserve. I went off for a 'Zubr' or 'bison' beer at an outdoor café by the empty parking lot and waited for my guide to arrive.

Mitek had the looks of a rural man of the earth, a round, ruddy face and a short, stocky body. He was dressed in a zipped green fleece jacket and a matching green felt peaked cap. We drove from the park office around the western edge of the park perimeter to a tall, square-beamed gate with 'Park Narodny' in wooden letters above it surrounded by wooden tiles. A man on a bicycle was leaving and they chatted. Walking on into the park, Mitek explained the man was the park's veterinarian. Damn! I should have told Mitek my profession.

Within the park I sensed an almost immediate change in Mitek. From the man simply earning a living by taking a tourist on a walk emerged a man who knew the ever-increasing joy at being at one with the natural world around him. He pointed out a black woodpecker as I had seen in Holland, a white-backed woodpecker, greater and lesser spotted woodpeckers. He knew exactly where they were but he was also constantly looking, listening, thinking. He reminded me of my dog when she's in the same kind of place and that's a compliment: vibrant, alert, animated, alive. Mitek's reward came as much from just being in the forest as it did from my paying him to guide me through it. He lived for the slow gradients of the country rather than the instant gratification of the city. I envied him.

He was also an encyclopaedic source of information. The blackbird alarm sound I heard was similar to the sound a predatory pine marten makes, he explained. He recognised woodpeckers from the sound of their knocking and showed me a hole made by a three-toed woodpecker. Hundreds of twitchers had come the spring before to see the bird. I learned that daphnia can act as a laxative, that new lime trees—lindens as he called them—grow off an old lime tree's root system.

He showed me where a greater spotted woodpecker had embedded spruce cones in the bark of a lime tree to provide winter food and how a hollow lime is an ideal habitat for a variety of animals including pine martens. There are 30 wolves in the park, he told me, that form and reform into packs. Sometimes they congregate into three packs but on other occasions they break up into five units. Behaviourists think there are two young males that will eventually emerge as alpha-males and that the five packs will become a permanent arrangement.

In this natural forest, where trees must vie with each other to reach the light at the canopy, species I think of as moderate and round in shape grow extraordinarily lean and tall. Maples were 40 metres high. So too were Scots pine. The lime trees were so imposing I thought they were oaks until I looked closer. From amongst them, both wrens chirped and woodpeckers tapped. I have never heard so much unremitting wood tapping.

Where beetles and flies congregated there were stinkhorn mushrooms, but that was not the only afternoon odour. Everywhere there was the sweet smell of decomposing wood. Late in our walk Mitek stopped. I put my finger on my camera's shutter button but he signalled me not to raise my camera. He smelled something. We stood, as rigid as statues, and he sniffed the air then pointed with a turn of his head to my left. I saw nothing. There was nothing, but then a wild boar came into view, followed by another. That is what he smelled.

We counted seven in the group, including a small one, a late-summer birth. For five minutes they snorted and rooted in the damp soil, oblivious to us standing only 12 metres away. Mitek gave me permission to raise my camera and as I did their ears perked, they looked at us and disappeared.

'They caught a reflection from your camera,' he explained.

Throughout the day, Mitek took photos—more than I did—mostly of mushrooms. They had not been here on his last visit and were an exciting addition, subterranean armies pushing out of the ground. Fungi have always given taxonomists problems. Are they plants or are they animals? The present compromise says they are neither and gives them their own kingdom status separate from plants and animals.

Mushrooms are the most familiar fungi but fungi vary from single celled micro-organisms or yeasts, some of which help raise flour, others of which infect dog's ears, through to moulds such as penicillin or forest slime to transient soft-bodied mushrooms or perennial, hard-bodied bracket fungi. Then there are lichens, like those covering the forest floors I've tramped throughout Scandinavia and the Baltics, symbiotic combinations of algae and fungi.

The plant algae part of the lichen are responsible for photosynthesis while the fungal element of the lichen takes minerals from the ground and provides a skeleton. Although they are part-plant, lichens are classified in the fungi kingdom. Around us, in late-September, the forest floor in Białowieża was a carpet of fungi, tube mushrooms such as boletes and many varieties of gill mushrooms—toadstools, parasols, honey mushrooms. On trees were countless colourful bracket fungi with hard chitinous perennial bodies. Mitek explained that bracket fungus from hardwood trees was once used as tinder, kept together with flint and a piece of metal for striking fires. Local bee-keepers used another kind of bracket fungus to smoke bees away from hives while they collected honey.

That afternoon was my first opportunity to talk extensively with a local man and as we walked I

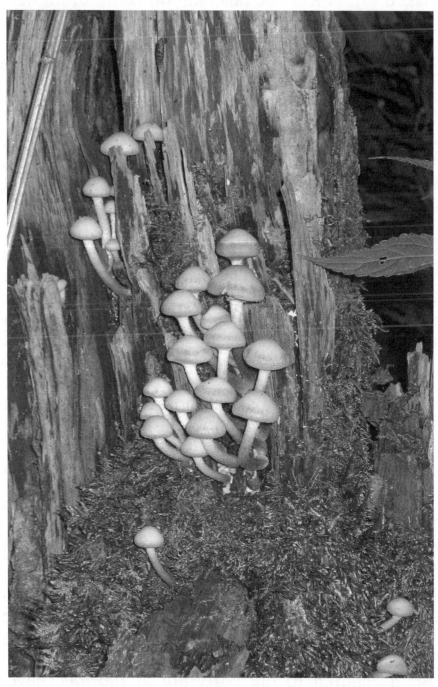

FUNGI GROWING ON A TREE TRUNK IN THE FOREST
AT BIAŁWIEŻA

asked Mitek why the farming was so different here in eastern Poland to that which I had seen in the Baltic states.

'Gomólka recognised, he accepted, that Polish peasant farmers would use passive resistance to prevent collective farms so there are none here,' he told me.

'In this part of Poland he allowed family farms to remain. However, in "new Poland"—in Prussia and Silesia and Pomerania—he created collective farms. When the government changed in 1989, these collective farms were ransacked of all their equipment. Friends of those who were now in power bought the collective farm lands and the collective workers with them. These people, living on the collectives, depended on the new landowners for their homes and their income. They were paid very low wages, some of them two złotys an hour.'

Mitek, who is a Baptist minister, was willing to talk about religion and nationalism.

'The corruption of the early 1920s has been repeated in recent times,' he said. 'In 1921 under Russian occupation, if you had soft hands or had two cows or if you sounded educated you were deported to the gulag.'

Thirty years later in the 1950s, Mitek was raised not under Russian occupation but certainly under its effective control. I'm sure that the fear of invasion from Russia remains elemental here on the frontier.

'Cardinal Wyszyński never relinquished control of the church to the Party but at the local level there was a closeness of church authorities and politicians. It was jobs for the boys. This part of

Poland is very mixed. There is less fanaticism. This is the type of toleration that is needed throughout Poland. In Belarus,' he added, 'if you are a Baptist they think you must be a spy for America.'

*   *   *

That evening I found a campsite close to the Belarus border to park in which was closed for the season. My telephone was picking up a signal and I phoned Julia to tell her how both of us were and that we both missed her. After sunset two heavily tattooed, shaven-headed, moustached East German Hell's Angels in a battered old Volkswagen bus joined us in the campsite for the night.

CARP IN WHITE WINE
Cut an onion in slices and lay the slices on the bottom of a pan.
Cut a carp fillet into slices and lay these on the onion.
Pour in half a bottle of an unoaked white wine (I used a New Zealand Sauvignon Blanc) and an equal amount of water.
Add salt, pepper and some lemon peel (I'd have added bay leaves if I'd had some).
Gently bring to a boil and, after skimming off the scum, cover and simmer on the lowest heat for 90 minutes.
If you're in a motorhome, turn off the fire alarm as, somehow, this cooking process makes it go manic.
After 90 minutes, remove the fish slices and reduce the remaining stock by simmering the pan

uncovered.

Cover the carp slices in stock and eat hot.

Refrigerate the remainder. The stock forms a firm jelly and the fish is even tastier cold the next day.

Sleep with all windows open and never, ever cook fish in a motorhome again.

*   *   *

The weather had favoured us from the start. It was yet another clear, sunny day. Macy dug vigorously in the fresh mole mounds throughout the campsite and after breakfast we returned to explore an unrestricted part of the forest. Mitek had been an excellent guide the previous day and I was now seeing things I hadn't noticed before.

The wych and European white elms were growing in damp, fertile soil. So too was an ash tree, almost 30 metres high, and almost a metre in diameter at its base. Mitek had told me that there's a Polish folk belief that ash leaves left under the bed sheets prevent marriage arguments. As a contingency I wanted to pick some but the leaves on this tree were too high for me to reach.

There was fruit ripe on the red elder and birds had been feasting. Here too, just as in the strict reserve, the oak trees were rigidly straight, almost 40 metres high, with lofty branches. At the edge of the forest by open meadows were willow and black alder. Mitek explained that alder was used for smoking meat and giving it its tint. The Norway spruce, some of which were even taller than the oaks, had crowns high in the forest canopy and visible root systems that were easy to trip over.

These—especially the diseased ones—were the woodpeckers' favourite trees, for foraging for insects. Hazels everywhere were shooting from old trees. I think the rake Macy found is probably made from a hazel shoot. Hazel is near perfect for making farm utensils such as pitchforks, spades and rakes.

We walked for six kilometres. I know how far because it was from the village to the game reserve and then back. There were hornbeam used for charcoal production and mountain ash used to flavour vodka, and more magnificent lime trees whose spring flowers produce a bounty of nectar for honeybees. The fresh forest smells on an early autumn morning were exhilarating to me but more provocative to Macy. Suddenly her tail rose erect and her nose went super-active but, learning from Mitek, I too could smell wild boar and I reined her in and leashed her to me. Returning along the same three-kilometre path was like walking a different journey. It was less than two hours later but as light moved higher in the canopy it now shone down to the ground and I felt as though I was on a different walk in a different forest. I understood how Mitek could never tire of taking visitors through the strict reserve.

*   *   *

The European wild horse or Tarpan no longer exists. The last remaining wild one, a mare, fell down a crevasse and died in 1880 at Askania Nove in the Ukraine while trying to escape capture. Seven years later the last Tarpan in captivity died in Munich Zoo. At the nearby Białowieża Reserve,

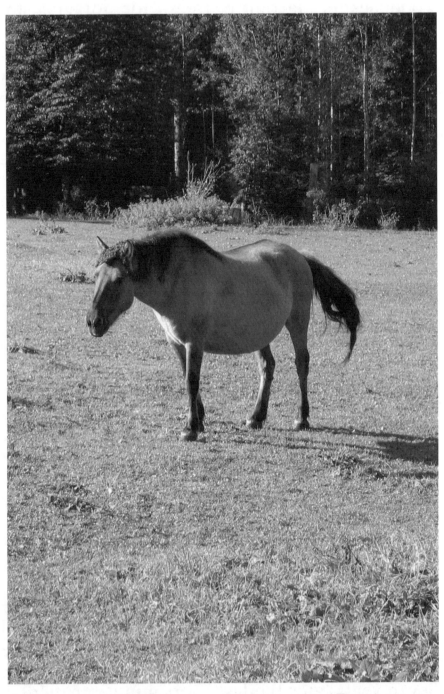

A 'DOMESTIC' TARPAN AT BIAŁOWIEŻA RESERVE

however, there are horses called 'domestic Tarpans' and I was curious to see them, as well as the other large mammals that inhabited this region which are also maintained in herds at the reserve.

Medieval farmers disliked Tarpans because they ate their crops and stole their domestic mares but, although Tarpans are extinct, there were also small domestic horses in eastern Poland. Some—very few—shared the Tarpan's dun-coloured coat and dorsal stripe, an idiosyncrasy caused by having an upright mane in which there is a mix of dark and light hairs. These ponies were called Bilgoraj Koniks.

In 1936 a professor at Poznan University, Tadeusz Vetulani convinced his government to confiscate all Koniks with blue-dun features for use in a breeding programme to perpetuate these visible characteristics. The Koniks were brought here to Białowieża and by 1939 there were 18 blue-dun coloured, dorsal-striped horses in the reserve.

Białowieża has been a private hunting ground for Lithuanian dukes, Russian tsars, Polish kings, Belarusian princes and more recently German Nazis. In the 1940s it was Hermann Goering's private hunting ground. Back in Sweden I had shared a ferry trip to Gotland with Hilmar-Lutz Poser, whose grandfather was veterinarian at the Berlin Zoo. His grandfather's boss was Lutz Heck who wrote, *Animals My Adventure.*

In the 1930s, Lutz Heck at the Berlin Zoo, and his brother Heinz Heck at the Hellabrunn Zoo in Munich embarked upon a selective horse-breeding programme but their claims were more audacious than Professor Vetulani's. They were, they claimed, not simply perpetuating a colour and form, mere morphological characteristics, but reviving the pure Teuton horse described in the *Nibelungenlied*. In *Animals My Adventure*, Lutz Heck claims, 'We succeeded in bringing back into existence . . . the primeval wild horse or Tarpan.'

Lutz Heck thought that looks alone were all that mattered and put his theory in simple terms, 'No animal can be extinct whose heritable constitution still exists. This constitution may be crossed with other species of animals, it may have suffered changes through race formations, but it still lives, and with the aid of our present-day knowledge of heredity it can be brought back as a whole.'

Using Polish Konik, Swedish Gotland, Icelandic, Nordic Forest, and Dartmoor mares, he bred them with Przewalski stallions and, 'brought back into existence . . . the wild horse.' Of course, he was doing no more than what Professor Vetulani in Poland was doing, merely perpetuating the looks of the Konik but using a wider range of European horses to do so.

The first animals to be seen on entering the Białowieża reserve are the Tarpan's domesticated relatives, the Koniks, descendants of Heck's breeding programme. Only 110–130 centimetres high, their grey colour is similar to the cattle I had seen in the Baltic states and here in north-eastern Poland. Genetically, blue dun is really dilute black and these horses had black manes, tails, legs and dorsal lines.

The Suffolk Wildlife Trust uses a few Polish Koniks to browse and graze through fen which has been left unmanaged for years, opening up land on which other grassland animals and plants can settle. So does the Lake Pape Nature Reserve in

Latvia where over 50 thrive, but both are insignificant compared to the 2500 Polish Koniks used to graze the Oostvaarderplassen Reserve in the Netherlands.

There was also a wolf enclosure surrounded by electric fencing and two red deer enclosures. There are 1500 red deer in the national park and the impressive males were coming into rut, roaring incessantly as I walked by. The males weighed 200 kilograms and grew new antlers each spring.

Deeper into the reserve were enclosures of '*zubronie*', the curious looking deep-chested dark-haired bison-domestic cow crosses, unique to Białowieża. The first generation hybrids are larger and heavier than their parents but only the females in that generation are fertile. Beyond the *zubronie* were little roe deer, weighing no more than whippets. There are 1000 of them in the park, as well as 1000 wild boar of which I'd seen seven the previous day.

Two thousand years ago European bison roamed all the way from western Europe to Siberia but by the seventeenth century the last remaining herds were in the protected hunting reserves here in Białowieża Forest. Białowieża was their last natural home. In *Animals My Adventure*, Heck writes that at the end of World War One there were 750 European bison in this forest but 'after the withdrawal of the German occupying force from the forests of Białowieża, hunters from the surrounding villages shot bison after bison in what had become no man's land, and soon there were only five bison left. And then came the news that on 28 February 1921 a poacher had killed the last survivor in that immemorial forest.'

That was the year that the new Polish government declared a large section of the forest a national park. The government also declared that it would repopulate the forest with bison by breeding from those in captivity in European zoos.

At the reserve there are two large meadows housing a selection of European bison but the story they tell here is different from that told by Lutz Heck. By the mid-nineteenth century, according to park publications, there were fewer than 1900 European bison in Poland and their numbers were declining. In 1915, there were only 785 animals left.

According to Białowieża Park information, when German troops occupied the forest in World War One it was they who killed 600 of these animals for their meat and hides. A concerned German scientist brought the slaughter to the attention of his government but by the time the German army retreated there were nine animals left in Białowieża. Within a few years all of these were shot by local poachers.

Whoever's history is true, a survey in 1923 found there were 54 European bison in Europe's zoos. The Society for the Protection of European bison was formed, two cows were brought from Sweden and a bull from Germany and the first calf was born here the following year. During World War Two, the forest was occupied first by the Russians and then by the Germans, but now both protected the small herd of breeding animals, posting signs saying poachers would be killed.

Enough survived for breeding to be resumed and some were released into the park in 1952. Now there are 3200 European bison living in the wild throughout Europe, 250 of them here in the park. Mitek explained to me that all of them descend from 12 animals and that 80 per cent—over 2500 of them—descend from just two individuals.

*   *   *

Aurochs are the ancestors of modern cattle. At one time they ranged from India to western Europe. At the Arsenal Museum in Stockholm, in the Livrustkammaren, there's a horn from one of the last aurochs, mounted in a silver setting. It is a trophy from Sochaczew, Poland from 1621, given to the Swedish king, who at that time was the prevailing regional power. The last surviving auroch died in Poland in 1627. Lutz Heck claimed he recreated this extinct species too. He certainly released animals he called aurochs into Białowieża Forest when, as he writes, 'the latter region, so uniquely suited to this purpose, came for about five years under German administration.'

Using the same method he'd used with the Tarpan ponies, Lutz and his brother Heinz simply crossbred existing varieties of cattle. Using Corsican, Scottish, Hungarian, Spanish and French animals he created a bovine Labradoodle but imbued it with mystical Teutonic qualities. He must have been a godsend to the Nazi authorities as he recreated these 'racially pure' ancestors of modern livestock, cattle known today simply and accurately at 'Heck's cattle'.

There's a chilling symmetry to some of Lutz's activities. In *Animals My Adventure* he writes movingly of the mental and physical torment of the animals at his Berlin Zoo: 'It seemed incredible,' he wrote in 1952, 'that a zoological garden with its innocent animals could be seriously considered as a target for bombs.'

In September 1939 the Germans had bombarded Warsaw's Zoological Gardens, killing Kasia the elephant, the giraffes, apes and antelopes. Within days of Warsaw's surrender Lutz Heck arrived at the zoo. He was responsible for all animal reserves in the Third Reich and arranged for Tuzinka, Kasia's two-year-old calf to be sent to Königsberg, the camels and llamas to Hanover, the hippopotamuses to Nuremberg, the Przewalski horses to Vienna, the lynxes and zebras to Schorfheide. From Białowieża he took the European bison and Professor Vetulani's Konik horses for himself.

Jan Zabinski who had been director of the Warsaw Zoo since 1929, and his wife Antonina, had known Heck personally before the war. Emptied of animals, the zoo was used for raising pigs, but the Zabinskis acquired another species for their empty zoo—desperate Jews. Mostly academics and professionals, they arrived by a subterranean passage in the former lion's enclosure. The Zabinskis obtained false identity papers for those whose appearance allowed them to be smuggled over to 'Aryan' Warsaw. Thirty people, too Jewish in looks to leave, remained hidden at the zoo until the war ended. In 1965 the Zabinskis were honoured by Israel, as Sugihara had been honoured, as 'Righteous Amongst the Nations'.

After the war Lutz Heck wrote, 'One of the most shocking chapters in the history of our day is that concerned with the almost complete destruction of a whole great species, full of vitality, simply through human folly and greed, ambition and blind destructiveness.' He was writing about the American bison.

Leaving the nature reserve I bumped into the campsite Hell's Angels from Groß Muckrow in former East Germany, who were buying honey from one of the souvenir stands. When we'd met the night before and failed to communicate because of the language barrier, I had one of them write down 'Groß Muckrow' and point it out on my map. I'd thought he was swearing about my dog. *'Nicht arbeit,'* one of them had explained, meaning either their old Beetle bus didn't work or they didn't. Now these Zapata-moustached, shaven-headed, gold-earringed, wrinkle-faced, leather-clad, piercing-blue eyed, pierced-skinned, guttural Germans were here to visit the animals at the zoo. Isn't that nice?

*   *   *

At the national park office I'd picked up a brochure for the 'Bison Track Path', a trail that tightly hugs the Belarus border, north of the park. Macy was bored of being jailed in the vehicle all morning and this was a great chance to see bison in the wild and give her some exercise, so with Barry's help I drove the circuitous 40 kilometre route to Narewka and with Mace on her lead went looking for the trail.

Green trail-markers took me through pine and spruce forest to a bridge over the Narewka River and the entrance to the park. Of course, dogs were prohibited. I'd passed other trails heading north and backtracked, hoping to go around the top of the park and connect with the bison trail as it left the park. Only a short portion of it is inside the park itself.

The landscape changed to birch and alder and then, by the stream's flood-plain, to willow shrubs and poplar. A bridge took me over the stream to some anonymous farm buildings and the trail turned right—the direction in which I wanted to travel—through young oak woodlands. There it ended, where another small stream joined the Narewka. And there was a beaver, sitting in the reeds, staring at me. There was no dam in sight, no beaver den, no signs of beaver-induced carnage, just a piggy-eyed, gormless little beaver, sitting, doing nothing. Macy hadn't noticed and I quietly called her to me and leashed her in but as I did so, the beaver casually turned, wiggled down to the water and swam leisurely away.

I decided to abort the bison hunt and hit the road back west towards Bielsk Podlaski where I'd be able to turn south without colliding with Belarus. As I bounced along the rutted road, jammed between lorries, I noticed a tick walking on my left leg, grabbed it and tossed it out the window. Five minutes later I saw one sunning itself on my right knee. I'd treated Macy so now, as far as the ticks were concerned, I was the best dish left on the menu; regardless of how messy the shower made the campervan I'd have to use it and then carry out a full body inspection that night. Besides, the smell of wild boar seemed to linger in the Roadtrek and I think it was coming from me.

*   *   *

Simonas had made me wary of Lukoil, the Russian chain of petrol stations, so I filled up at a Norwegian Statoil and amused myself by trying to guess the philosophies of the politicians on electoral posters that had sprouted everywhere. It was tough as they all seemed to follow the same set of rules.

1. Don't smile. This is a serious business. Try to ooze testosterone.
2. Wear a red-and-white tie. You don't want voters to think you're not a nationalist.
3. Grow a bushy moustache. Try to be a subliminal Lech Walesa but under no circumstances let your moustache remind voters of The Village People. If you look like you're gay, you're dead in the water.
4. Look po-faced. Don't even give away a glimmer of the fact that you want to get your hands in the pork barrel.
5. Don't be a woman because they don't ooze testosterone and should be home having patriotic Polish babies but if you are, have your teeth whitened and wear a red and-white-dress.

There was more who-gives-a-shit tarmac on the road to Lublin. There are no E roads in this part of Poland so there's no EU money for improvements. Don't get me wrong. I'm not complaining about the scenery. What's so attractive about these unimproved roads is that they still go through every town and village in the region. Church spires on this flat plain dominated the vista, announcing where each town was and whether it was Catholic, Orthodox or both. Of course, for centuries this region, from Białystock to Lublin was also Jewish, often predominantly so.

Each town or village had a full inventory of rustic wooden homes but there was also a heroic amount of new building going on, especially of homes. The trucks I was jockeying with on the road were makes that were unknown to me: Jelcz, Star, Autosan, Kamaz, Zul, Steyr, Tatra, Liaz. Scanias and Volvos were rare. South of Lublin there was suddenly a pristine, single mile stretch of brand new motorway and Macy relaxed, but, although I had now hooked on to the E road from Warsaw to L'viv in the Ukraine, the road surface soon reverted to 'Polish regular' and we bounced along, on one occasion so badly that I broke a tail-light suspended from the rear bumper.

At Lublin the Great European Plain ended and now I was in a gently rolling agricultural landscape, not quite hilly, but almost. Corn was being cropped with sparkling new equipment while the hop fields had already been harvested. Large herds of cattle grazed on both sides of the road. It was a pastoral and appealing scene. There was mistletoe on the trees and flash black BMWs and Mercs with Ukrainian plates whizzing past on the roads. The familiar and the unexpected.

*   *   *

Zamość is an absolute jewel, an original Italian Renaissance town with a glorious, 100 square metre piazza surrounded by exquisite houses with richly decorated pastel facades over columned

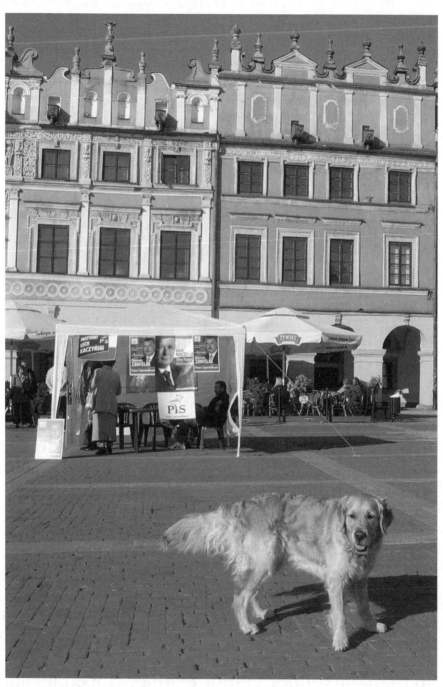

THE BEAUTIFUL ITALIANATE PIAZZA AT ZAMOŚĆ

arcades, built by wealthy merchants. Alleys lead off from the corners of the piazza but also from the centre of each side so that the houses stand in individual groups of four. Surrounding the square is a symmetrical grid of streets and beyond that grid, fortifications: high defensive bastions. This was one of the few Polish towns not destroyed in the seventeenth-century war with Sweden—the so-called 'Swedish Deluge'—and more by luck than anything else, although there were heavy battles in the region, subsequent wars passed the city by. It was even spared in World War Two.

Count Zemoyski was a local landowner who in the eighteenth century kept a herd of Tarpans at his nearby private zoological park, and was a descendent of the Count Zemoyski who was head of the army of the Polish-Lithuanian Commonwealth in the sixteenth century. His land was on the commercial trade route connecting northern and western Europe with the Black Sea ports and Zemoyski commissioned an Italian architect from Padua, Bernardo Morando, to create the perfect Renaissance town. Zamość soon attracted traders—Scots, German, Hungarian, Italian and Greek but especially Armenians and Jews—who settled here.

I parked outside the walls of the old town and under a cloudless blue sky we strolled into the piazza which Macy cleared quickly of pigeons. In front of me to the left at the top of the square was the copper-topped pink tower of the Town Hall with a double, fan-shaped stone stairway leading up to the first floor entrance. Macy zipped up and down the stairs to the amusement of the very few people, mostly schoolchildren, who were in the square.

Restaurants had set up tables with umbrellas in the corners of the piazza and I sat in the sun at one on the north side for an amber 'Żywiec' beer, and hoped that Mace would follow her job description and pick up strangers. She didn't and, strangely, I wasn't in the mood for doing so for myself so we walked the arcade around the piazza, window-shopping. Many of the merchants' houses have been converted to offices or shops. To enter a shop we walked through high wooden doorways into vestibules and then right or left into one shop or another. I browsed 'antiques' in one shop while Macy got stroked and praised.

Outside each home was a plaque commemorating who had once lived there. Some were lived in by academics who taught at the academy Zamoyski had built behind the town hall. Some were the homes of Jewish traders—by the onset of World War Two, almost half the population of Zamość was Jewish. Most were the homes of Armenians.

The history of Armenians in Poland is as old as the history of Jewish settlement. They first arrived in great numbers in the fourteenth century, migrating, as the Jews often did, for commercial reasons. Like the Greeks and the Jews, the Armenians were cosmopolitan traders. By the Middle Ages there were over 200,000, mostly concentrated here in the south-east of the country. Like the Jews, they kept their language, style of dress, culture and religious beliefs intact.

Armenians in Poland lived in well-organised communities and just as Jewish communities were granted rights to have their own administrations—

the *'kahals'*—the Armenians has their *'voit'*. The Armenians initially traded with the East, carpets, jewellery, garments, leather, and evolved into manufacturing goods for the Polish market. The Armenian merchants' homes around the piazza were owned by families who had prospered.

When trade with the East declined in the eighteenth century, and the Polish Armenian Church had formed a union with the Polish Roman Catholic Church, many Armenians became estate owners and by the turn of the nineteenth century they had lost their language. All that remains of their Armenian origins are their Polish-influenced surnames: Apakanovics, Yakhowicz, Barovitch, Grigorovicz, Mrozianovsky, Malowski.

Some Armenians even became members of the *'szlachta'*—the most powerful Polish caste, those of noble blood. The *szlachta* were radically different from Western European aristocracy. While Western aristocracy derived its power from the emperor or king, in Poland the *szlachta* grew out of regional clans and came to govern virtually independent principalities of all sizes, from huge estates such as the Zemoyskis' down to areas that were no more than local farms. Their pride in who they were meant that it was beneath them to carry on business. Instead they employed Jews to run their mills, stills and inns, and to act as their financiers.

The former editor of the *New York Times Book Review*, and author of *Shtetl, The History of a Small Town and an Extinguished World*, Eva Hoffman, quotes a late-sixteenth-century Venetian envoy, Pietro Duodo: 'There are many Calvinists and Lutherans (in Poland), but most numerous are the

Jews; because the nobility is ashamed of trade, the peasants are too backward and oppressed, and the burghers too lazy, the entire Polish trade is in Jewish hands. The aristocrats treat them with respect, because they have profits from them, the government treats them so, because when in need, it can extract great sums from them.'

In some regions of Poland the *szlachta* made up 20 per cent of the population. They addressed each other as *'Pan'* or *'Pani'*—'Sir' or 'Madam'. At a restaurant in London I once asked a Polish waiter whether, as is common in the United States and Canada, the gold ring bearing an elaborate crest that he wore was his university ring. He explained it was his family coat of arms. The *szlachtas'* consciousness of their special identity has survived three partitions of the country, the total abolition of the state and, in the twentieth century under Communism, the abolition of their caste. Families such as the Poniatowskis continue to participate in state affairs and one aspect of their noble culture has survived: today, all Poles address each other as *'Pan'* or *'Pani'*.

*　　　*　　　*

In World War Two, this region of Poland was chosen by the Germans for colonisation. The black soil is fertile and this was the exact type of territory that they wanted for *'lebensraum'*, for 'living room'. Over 100,000 people were removed from Zamość and the surrounding villages. The Jews were murdered, the Poles of Armenian descent were 'relocated' and German settlers brought in to what was renamed *'Himmlerstadt'*. At the end of the

297

war, the German settlers were in turn killed or driven away and the Poles returned but within a few years, under pressure from Russia, large sections of the regional population were dispersed once more.

At a grocery store on one of the cobbled streets behind the piazza I bought herring, a bundle of thin, smoked sausages, eggs and onion buns then headed west for Roztoczański National Park where I planned to stay for the night. The road went through Szczebrzeszyn, the most difficult to pronounce town in all of Poland, and at the western end of the town square was an imposing building that could only ever have been a grand, brick synagogue. The sign on the building said, '*Dom Kultury*'.

I parked and, with Macy, walked the narrow residential streets on the hills behind. Fenced dogs wanted to attack Macy but small ones who trotted about loose were intrigued by the blonde city chick and came over to scent her out. Locals smiled and talked to me when they saw these encounters but, alas, I didn't understand a word. At the top of the first hill was a street sign, '*Ul Cmentarna*'. The synagogue's cemetery must be nearby. It took another quarter hour before, climbing a forested hill at the top of that street, I saw a fallen tombstone.

During the Soviet era cemeteries were subject to a campaign of oblivion. They were an obstacle to the Soviet rewriting of history. In this one the overgrowth of vegetation was so profuse that shrubs and bushes had become trees. Very recently, certainly within the last two months, the overgrowth had been cut back and paths created around the stones, many of which had fallen and could only be discerned by the perfect rectangles of green moss that covered them. Some were still standing at crooked angles.

Using my fingers and the palm of my hand I rubbed and lifted away the thick verdant green moss from one of the fallen stones and saw underneath a pair of beautifully carved delicate hands raised in prayer. It must have been the gravestone of a woman. I looked for dates, but all the writing was in Hebrew, even the numbers. Some of the stones were impressively grand, both in the hewing of the stone itself and in the carving, while others looked as if they were simply natural stones that had writing inscribed on them. In the fading light I took photographs to bring back and have translated for me:

'Here is buried an honest man. Old and full of days he walked on the perfect way and cleaved to the true righteous people. Menachem Yaakov. Died the 2nd of Chanukah 5676. May his soul be bundled in the bundle of life.'

'Here is buried a man with a good name, died on the eve of Sabbath, the 29th Shevat. From the beginning an honest man, willed by love of just people and his deeds are worthy. He sat in his tent and busied himself with Torah. He made the poor happy. He got up hurriedly to bring them in and to give meals. He received guests with love and happiness. With a nice expression he fed them generously. With presents he supported them with his outstretched hand. His wisdom and understanding were great. Happy with his portion was his soul. Rabbi Menachem Mendel. May his memory be a blessing. May his soul be bundled in the bundle of life.'

It dropped below freezing the night I camped at Roztoczański National Park and I missed my hot-water bottle—she was back in London. The park's symbol is the Konik pony, as we were near Bilgorai, where Count Zemoyski kept the last true herd of small wild horses. I turned the heat on in the camper, dressed in hat, gloves and scarf and took Macy for a 6 a.m. walk through frost-covered grass into the adjacent pine forest. When we returned and she tried to drink from her water bowl she discovered it had frozen solid overnight.

To the sound of Tina Turner on the local radio station, I headed south on anonymous back roads. The free-ranging dogs pottering by the road were always small, even those trotting or running in packs behind horse-drawn carts or tractors. South of the E road connecting Krakow to L'viv, the land took on a gentle roll. Vernacular architecture was different, the mortar between the squared logs of old homes often painted—usually white but also in pastel colours. This land, Galicia, where my mother's grandmother was born, was annexed to the Austro-Hungarian Empire after the First Partition of Poland in 1772 and did not return to Polish rule until the country was created once more after World War One. *Baedeker's Austria-Hungary* (1911) suggests giving the region a miss.

'In the small towns and in the country the inns are generally primitive and dirty; they are usually kept by Jews.' The guide explains that in 'Cracow,

300

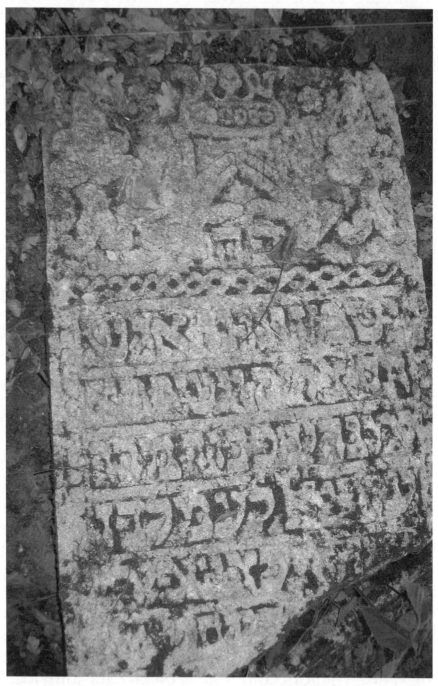

A JEWISH GRAVESTONE HIDDEN IN THE
UNDERGROWTH AT SZCZEBRZESZYN

Lemberg and Czernowitz German is understood by all the cultured inhabitants so a knowledge of Polish is unnecessary.' If travelling by train from Cracow to Czernovitz, the train goes through, 'Tarnow, a town of 37,276 inhabitants (half of them Jews),' then Rzeszow, 'with 26,840 inhab. (half Jews),' on to 'Lember, Polish Lwow, French Leopol, the capital of Galicia, with 206, 575 inhab. (11 per cent Jews),' then through 'Stanislau—a busy trading town with 33,000 inhab. (more than half Jews),' to 'Czernowitz (Bucharest), 86,870 (about one third Jews).'

I stopped at a farmers' market in the town of Dynow where I bought three massive beefsteak tomatoes, end-of-season raspberries, a bunch of chives and some beets. On the pavement outside the market there was a row of elderly women selling cheese. I bought a kilo of fresh-made cottage cheese from a kindly looking lady in a blue wool jacket and formal Black Watch tartan skirt; the cheese had formed into the shape of the bag it was in.

At a nearby bakery I bought several buns that looked like deep-crust pizzas sprinkled with crispy onions but tasted a zillion times better. In the village of Urzjoyice, outside almost every home lining the road were vegetable stands and I bought cabbage, onions, red peppers and more potatoes. Each home was surrounded by wire fences, probably to keep their dogs in, and in the gardens, the remaining flowers were all straining towards the sun. On these roads the only other traffic was bicycles, tractors, old Fiat Polski cars and local trucks.

The rolling landscape gradually turned into

proper, undulating hills and Macy's disapproval of rough, potholed roads became evident. She crawled under my legs for security. I drove through a meandering valley where a narrow-gauge railway line twisted and turned along the bank of the San river, then up into the hills and looked down into the next valley, where the homes looked like liquorice allsorts spattered on the hillsides leading down to the river below. Over the next crest and into the next valley where there were squared-beam, log houses, cud-chewing cows and scurrying chickens. Now the hilltops were covered in trees. In a valley I pulled off the road and we walked past a man and his pony ploughing perfect furrows in his field, to a swaying suspension footbridge over the river. Wagtails dived then ascended in unison like a pack of Stuka fighters.

There's a brilliant open-air museum near the hilltop town of Sanok—the Museum of Folk Architecture, a *'skansen'*, as ethnographic museums are generically called in Polish, named after the first of their type at Skansen in Stockholm. The tourist season had ended and there were no guided tours in English, but the English language guidebook explained where the farmhouses, inns, churches, windmills, animal parlours, stately homes, subsistence hovels, schoolhouses, even town houses came from. All the region's ethnic groups were represented, the hill dwellers, the valley dwellers, the Catholics, the Orthodox, the smaller ethnic groups such as Ukrainian Boykos and Lemkos.

Up until 65 years ago, half of the inhabitants of this region were Jewish but their presence is omitted at the Sanok *skansen*. As at every

303

ethnographic museum I visited in the Baltic states and Poland that reality, that intense presence, is absent from the modern telling of local history. The difficult past is avoided and replaced by fantasy.

The cliff-top town of Lesko, south-east of Sanok, is the gateway to the Bieszczady, a remote south-eastern finger of Poland that sticks like a disapproving left-handed 'thumbs down' into the adjacent Ukrainian province of Halychnya. Stubble in fields was being burned as I drove by, nourishing the land for the next harvest. Logging trucks, each with six to eight massive logs on board, lumbered along the narrow roads up to this isolated town above the San river.

As in Sanok and elsewhere in this beautiful region of the old Austro-Hungarian province of Galicia, the Jewish community made up over half of the population. The imposing Spanish-looking Renaissance synagogue, with the Ten Commandments and a quotation from the Torah still legible on the front facade, was once an integral part of the town's defensive system. The building is now the 'galeria'—an art gallery. We walked down the steep hill beside the synagogue, dogs barking as Macy passed. At a wooded crossroad I turned left and Macy instantly trotted through a rusty open gate in the heavy undergrowth and up steep steps into a green, sun-dappled, sprawling, hilltop cemetery, as beautiful and evocative as any I have seen.

Lesko was settled 500 years ago by Spanish Jews fleeing the Inquisition and the Spanish heritage is evident, not only in the synagogue's architecture but in my mother's family's appearance. I don't

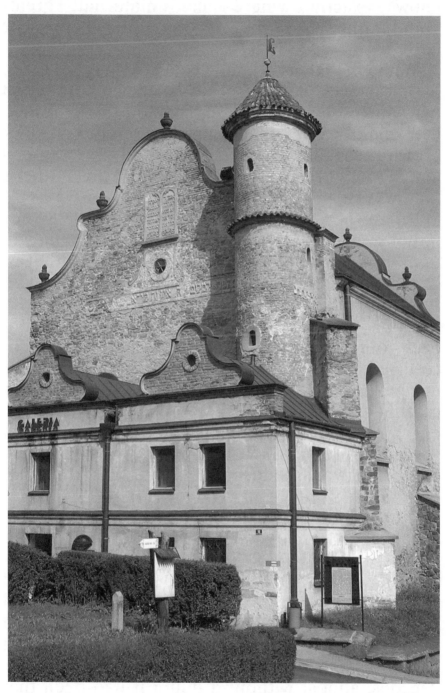

THE GALLERY AND OLD SYNAGOGUE IN LESKO

know exactly where my maternal great-grandmother lived but it was somewhere near here.

While my father's family is tall, with blue, green or hazel eyes, often freckle-faced with fiery red hair, my mother's family are smaller, fine featured, with round rather than long faces and dark, dark brown eyes and hair. I inherited my father's family's height and facial features and my mother's family's eye and hair colouring.

When they arrived in Canada in the 1880s they initially made a living as rag traders, dealing in '*shmattas*', a quintessentially Yiddish word that is, in fact, the Polish for rags. While Christians and Jews in this region of Europe maintained a spiritual separateness, their cultures influenced each other. Driving through Poland I bought cottage cheese similar to the type my mother tells me her mother made, and pickled herring, sour cream and local bread that, to me was '*challah*' or egg bread. I saw jars of beet borscht for sale in grocery stores and drove past carp farms. Who knows on which side of the divide chicken soup originated.

*   *   *

The cemetery we'd found was deeply forested and contained over a thousand ornately carved Baroque tombstones. One was deeply embedded in the trunk of a tree that was itself over a metre in diameter. The grounds had been abandoned for decades, almost without a doubt it had been that way since the early 1940s, when after almost 500 years of continuous residence, suddenly not a

306

single soul was left alive to tend the graves. Within the last three years, some trees were felled, saplings removed and the undergrowth contained in a gentle manner that added a serenity to the surroundings.

Macy and I were not the only ones visiting. Two young men and a woman, all in their very early twenties, were walking amongst the stone tablets, pausing, taking photographs. Macy introduced herself to them, allowing me to do so as well. They had been on a hiking holiday in Bieszczady National Park, and had stopped here on their way back to university in Krakow. All spoke English reasonably well.

They wanted to know how I had found such a remote place but that is, in fact what I wanted to learn from them. The woman, well-tanned, round-faced with her dark brown hair in a pony-tail, explained that they heard about this cemetery at university.

'It is a surprise. We thought that the Jews lived in cities. This is so peaceful. So beautiful.'

I asked what they learned at school of the Jewish heritage in Poland.

'It is different now,' she explained. 'My parents were told nothing but we learned about them. They were good in business. The Jews that survived the Nazis supported the Soviets. It is easy to understand why.'

I asked why they had stopped here and she explained, 'It is when you visit here that you see real people. They lived and they died and they were remembered. It is very moving. More Polish people should visit such a place as this.'

*   *   *

Only five years after the Germans purged this region of Jews, the Poles cleansed the region of its remaining non-Catholics—140,000 Ukrainians—by deporting them, the first tens of thousands to the Ukraine and then in 'Operation Wisła' the remaining people were dispatched to the new 'Recovered Territories' of western Poland, the former German states of Prussia, Silesia and Pomerania, that were given to the Poles by Stalin as war booty. The Ukrainians were to be scattered and assimilated into the Polish population.

The entire Bieszczady and Beskid Niski regions bordering the Ukraine and Slovakia were denuded of people. Buildings, and even churches, in the remaining ghost towns were disassembled board by board and removed. It was not only the local inhabitants who were transported. So too were their animals, although not often with the families. Few had time to collect their possessions. Most of these soil-tilling peasants were given less than three hours to collect a maximum of 25 kilograms of luggage per person and attend for deportation.

Most of the Ukrainians deported were from two distinctive groups, Boykos and Lemkos, mountain dwellers named after distinctive features of their speech. For two years at the end of World War One, there was an independent Lemko Republic in these mountains but in 1920 it was incorporated into the new state of Poland.

The term 'Ukrainian' is relatively new, a twentieth-century creation. For most of their history, 'Ukrainians' were 'Ruthenians'. Some people in the nearby western regions of what is

308

now the Ukraine continued to call themselves 'Ruthenians' until Stalin banned the term.

The Boykos are ethnic Ukrainians with a distinctive pattern of speech. Lemkos are also ethnic Ukrainians, their name derived from their unique use of an expression of speech, 'lem', meaning 'but' or 'only' or 'like'. In the Ukraine, both Boykos and Lemkos describe their ethnicity as 'Ukrainian'. In Poland, however, there is a rekindling of interest in their distinctive ethnic identity and a small but growing number of individuals in Poland are defining themselves ethnically as Lemkos. Andy Warhol is probably the most famous ever Lemko.

Boykos and Lemkos are mostly members of the Ukrainian Greek Orthodox Church. Driving from Lesko south-east to the remotest region of the Bieszczady I came across several freshly restored wooden Lemko three-domed churches, with the domes arranged in a line, the central dome larger than the others. The beautiful Lemko church at Horzow is now Roman Catholic.

The human suffering of these deportations was considerable but the consequences to the local environment were astounding. With people, livestock and domestic pets removed, the Bieszczady reverted to nature. Wildlife flourished—especially mammals—and within only a few years these mountains became a refuge for brown bears, lynx, wolves, elks, wild boar, red deer and roe deer. Hamsters migrating north from the Black Sea found ideal breeding grounds in the abandoned meadows. Today it is the UNESCO-recognised Eastern Carpathians World Biosphere Reserve. The lynx is the emblem of Bieszczady

National Park.

*   *   *

In the distance, in ever diminishing shades of blue were mountains, the first I had seen on my travels. There was a chill in the air and smoke funnelled from cottage chimneys even though it was only two in the afternoon. Most of the surrounding forest was Carpathian beech, just turning autumnal yellow. Amongst them were firs, sycamores and maples. Alders grow along the banks of the many streams.

The sky became overcast as I drove south. I had planned to go hiking with Macy, up to the 'poloniny', the bare, windswept mountain meadows where Boyko farmers grazed their sheep during the summer months for centuries, but now I had second thoughts. The weather could change in an instant and my mobile phone was not picking up signals even down at these relatively low levels.

A few miles past an ostrich farm (the last thing I would have expected to see in Poland), and outside Ustrzyki Górne but inside the boundaries of the park itself I gave a lift to two hitchhikers on their way to Wetlina. Ryszard's English was excellent. His girlfriend understood what we were saying but was too bashful to join in, passing comments to Ryszard for onward transmission to me. Ryszard thanked me for giving them a lift.

'You are far away from home. Why do you come here?' he asked. I explained I was interested in visiting parts of Europe that the British seldom come to and asked if he had visited Britain. He told me his younger brother was working 'in

310

England' at a restaurant in Fort William in Scotland but he had never visited. His girlfriend reminded him that they had visited the United States together.

'I like America. America is good friend. I like to work there but work visa is much money, $100.' When I asked why he wanted to work in the United States rather than elsewhere in the EU he explained that Europe didn't want him.

'We cannot work in Germany. Only Ireland and England. We are members of European Union but they treat us as not good enough. Germany wants to be our friend but I cannot work there. Russia wants to control us with economy. It is good decision we are friends with America.'

I asked him what he thought of Britain and Ryszard explained, 'England is OK.' His girlfriend nodded. 'England and Ireland is OK. Good countries. I feel good with England. Mr Blair. Mr Beckham. England is right. England treats us as equals.'

*   *   *

From Wetlina, rather than circling back up to Lesko I took a back road paralleling the Slovakian border and headed west into the hills towards the Low Beskids. I drove past an old man hand-scything a field while his wife gathered the cut grass by hand. At the top of one pass, amongst rolling pastureland I chanced on a large wooden pen of sheep surrounded by nine resting guard dogs. They were Tatra Mountain sheepdogs, quiet, thick-coated mastiffs.

One of them, a young tan-and-white male

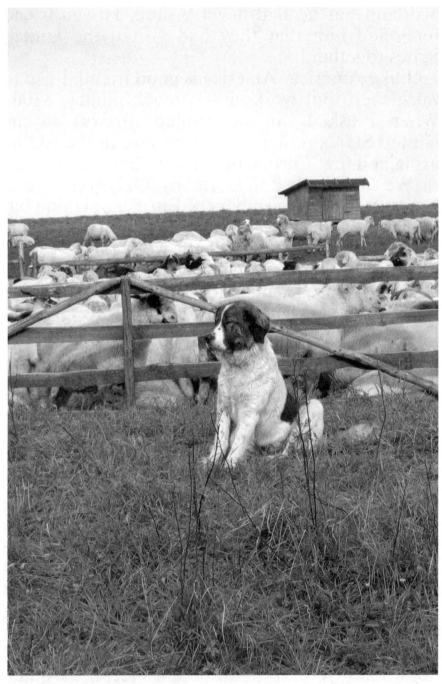

A Tatra Mountain sheepdog, guarding his flock

closest to me in front of the sheep pen had a severe limp. His right front leg was visibly swollen from the paw up to the elbow. My first thought was to examine it but he would have had my hand as an appetiser if I'd tried. Beyond him, to the side of the large pen were the eight other dogs, some creamy-white, others tan and white, brown and white, and black and white, lying in groups in the grass. They were here in large numbers because there are more wolves in the Bieszczady than anywhere else in the EU.

I took a few photos through the window of the Roadtrek but, when I opened the door, the limper went alert, sprang forward on his good leg and barked at me. Within seconds his cohorts were beside him, also barking at me, as frightening a canine display as I have seen. I retreated back into the Roadtrek and they stood there, between me and the sheep, until I drove off.

*   *   *

Here in the remote Eastern Carpathians wolves flourished, and were freed from the predations of farmers and hunters by the clearances carried out by the Polish government after World War Two. The clearances also meant that the wolves survived the predations of Communist Party planners, who were busy wiping out wolf populations elsewhere—there were no farmers and no livestock here, hence no need to waste resources on wolf eradication.

Relieved of human pressures, all wildlife flourished, especially deer—the wolf's favoured prey—and the wolf packs followed their seasonal migration. In the summer the packs rested in the highlands, on mountain ridges visited only by intrepid hikers, and would descend from their strategic vistas to attack their prey. As deer moved into the valleys for the winter the wolves followed them down, using forest roads in the winter.

During the Communist years, it was official policy to exterminate wolves and bears from both the Polish and Slovakian sides of the Carpathian mountains. That meant that the need for native, livestock guarding dogs such as the Tatra Mountain sheepdog and the almost identical Slovenský Čuvač, dropped. These breeds, together with their close relatives the Hungarian Kuvasz and Komondor, were now bred for companionship or show rather than utility. When farmers were allowed to return to this eastern region of Poland, where neither wolves nor brown bear had been eliminated, livestock, especially sheep, were prey once more.

A livestock guarding breed has a distinctive personality. Unlike herders such as Border collies, that stalk, chase and are naturally predatory, good livestock guards lack those characteristics. Raised from puppyhood with the flock, they are completely trustworthy and don't interfere with the routines of feeding, breeding or lambing. Like those I saw in Poland, they stay close to their charges, relaxed but attentive and they bark viciously when a predator appears, and place themselves between the flock and the threat, just as the limping dog did when I opened my vehicle's door.

The Carpathian wolf is a typically adaptive carnivore. A pack's usual hunting range covers around 45 square kilometres during the summer and twice that range in the winter. It's not unusual for a wolf to travel 20 kilometres in a day while stalking prey. In this region of Poland they also target wild boar.

During the summer, wild boar makes up around a quarter of their diet but during the winter this increases to almost half. Researchers know this because they analyse wolf droppings. Across the mountains in Slovakia, where swine fever—a highly infectious virus disease with devastating financial consequences to the pig industry—has transmitted to wild boar, preliminary findings show that the disease is not spreading where wild boar are predated on by wolves. As the wolves catch the weakest boars, they effectively weed out the most diseased boar before they can spread swine fever to the herd.

Although it may be controlling the spread of swine fever, the Carpathian wolf remains a villain in the region's folk memory. While the brown bear has been officially protected in Poland since 1957, it was not until 1998 that the wolf obtained similar protection. More than half of Poland's still meagre population of approximately 750 wolves are here in the Bieszczady mountains. From here, migration corridors have been created to allow them to mix with wolves successfully reintroduced into the Polish and Slovakian Tatra Mountains.

Stray, dispersing wolves from this region have made their way to the Czech Republic, Hungary, Austria and Germany where they have either been shot by hunters or been victims of road traffic accidents. Farmers, although compensated, say that wolves should be eliminated to avoid livestock losses from predation. Hunters say wolf hunting should be permitted to reduce deer losses from wolf predation. The wolf's best friends are urban voters.

*   *   *

I stopped by a narrow-gauge rail track to let Macy exercise in the woods. The adjacent church, Orthodox in style, was now Catholic. In the unkempt grounds around the church were multitudes of rusted Orthodox crosses but through a gate in the stone wall at the back of the church there was a second, immaculate cemetery where the oldest polished black headstone I found was dated 1947, the year the Lemkos were cleansed from the region.

A mile further up the dirt road another stream joined the one that ran alongside the road. In a copse were the remnants of another Orthodox cemetery, fallen crosses amongst shrubs and trees. There had once been a village here, but in 1947 all but the dead were removed.

At Komancza there were three churches, a triple onion-domed wooden Lemko Orthodox church—freshly restored—another wooden church at the opposite end of the village, built in the 1950s for the Catholic 'newcomers', and a large modern construction in the centre of the village for the Uniate majority.

Uniates are Catholics who incorporate many aspects of Orthodox tradition into their faith. Just north of Komancza, in this back end of oblivion is the place where the Communists kept Cardinal Stephan Wyszynski under house arrest in the 1950s

316

for opposing their rule. I camped nearby.

*   *   *

'Girl? Boy?' he asked and when I replied 'Girl,' he returned to his Ford Transit van, opened the door and released his youthful, longhaired German shepherd who bounded over to Macy, lifted her hindquarters with his long snout and checked out her hormonal status.

Just west of Komancza, the Bieszczady mountain range gives way to the Beskid Niski, or the Low Beskids. This is the historical divide between the East and West Carpathian Mountains. Further to the west, in the direction I was going, were the Tatra Mountains, the highest in the West Carpathians, as imposing as the Alps. Our campsite was a grassy field by a nature reserve and, until a German couple arrived later, the only other camper was Transit-man and his German shepherd.

He was in his late forties, balding, heavy set and he knew only a few bits of English, though obviously more words than I knew in Polish. On the wooden table beside his van was a large red plastic bowl filled with mushrooms. He caught my eye-line, pointed to the mushrooms and then to the forest-covered hills behind the campsite and said, 'Much'. I nodded. As I departed to take Macy for her exercise, he returned to me with an empty bowl and offered it to me, pointing once more to the forest.

We walked the trails in the hilly nature reserve for an hour and I picked the occasional mushroom I recognised, although I was more interested in simply keeping my foothold. The trails were steep and the ground unexpectedly wet. I returned to the campsite and made myself a simple supper: sectioned beefsteak tomatoes sprinkled with salt and olive oil, a large wedge of cottage cheese sprinkled with black pepper and a massive pile of late-season raspberries, all accompanied by a large onion bun, sliced open and spread with unsalted Polish butter. At the far side of the field, Transit-man lit a butane fire and fried his mushrooms in butter. When he finished he beckoned me over and offered me some.

This is an interesting situation. A stranger picks mushrooms, cooks them and offers them to you. You have no idea whether he knows the difference between edible and poisonous mushrooms. You do not speak a word of his language and he speaks six and a half of yours. You may die— uncomfortably—if you eat what is offered to you. It's a question of civility. Do you eat the mushrooms? I looked around and it was apparent he had been there for days. Living on mushrooms. He looked healthy. His dog was still alive and was being fed mushrooms too. So I ate them and they were absolutely delicious.

Macy and the young shepherd raced figure eights, tumbled, rolled and played. I went back to my camper and got a couple of Estonian beers from the fridge. He went to his camper and got an unlabelled bottle of paint stripper. We shared.

'Beer,' I said, giving him a can.

'*Pivo*,' he replied, meaning either 'Thanks' or 'Beer'.

'Vodka,' he said, sticking his chest out, looking smiling but stern as he handed me a yellow plastic mug he had partly filled. *'Nazdrovyeh,'* he added, raised his mug, and tossed it back, so I followed suit and was startled to realise that it didn't taste like paint stripper at all. It was really smooth and had the smell of fresh-cut hay. As I wiped a crust of onion bun around the remaining mushrooms from my plate, he offered me more of his vodka.

I'd forgotten that vodka isn't Russian, but Polish, originally distilled by Polish monks, for 'medicinal purposes'. *'Wodka'*, in Latin was *'aqua vitae'*, the 'water of life' and although it was originally made from rye, once potatoes became a common harvest they too were used to produce vodka. The most expensive Polish vodkas are distilled from special varieties of potatoes grown near the Baltic.

I don't know what Transit-man's vodka was distilled from but there's something earthy and basic and deeply rewarding in sitting outdoors on a crisp evening, with a jacket and scarf on, sharing stomach-warming mushrooms that have just been picked and fried in butter, and stomach-warming spicy vodka with someone with whom you share absolutely nothing but a meal and a common humanity.

*   *   *

At dusk a German camper van arrived and the following morning I met the occupants, a couple my age who had planned to stay in Bierszczady Park but decided to move on. They had dropped off their 26-year-old son at the Ukrainian border the day before and were going hiking for the next two weeks in Slovakia and Hungary before

319

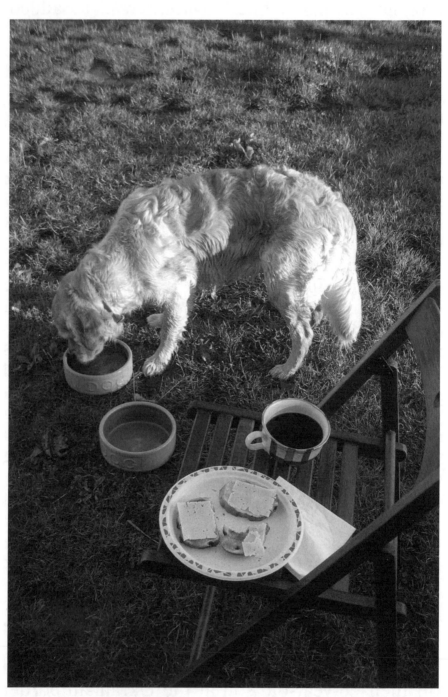

BREAKFAST FOR TWO

returning to pick him up. It was another freezing morning but cloudlessly sunny day. At dawn the only sounds were from the nearby tinkling brook. Birds, if they were present, were silent.

The longer I travelled in this region of Europe, the more I was coming to enjoy my intermittent chats with German campers. Those travelling in early autumn shared common characteristics. They were usually around my age, middle-class professionals and spoke English. This couple had recently visited Toronto where the woman's elderly uncle, a submariner in World War Two, lived. They had visited the Gaspésie region of Quebec the year before and told me they loved every minute of it and wanted to return some day.

The regions of Europe I had travelled through had been ravaged in living memory by Germans. There were reminders at every turn. An entire culture, one of the vital essences of this cosmopolitan continent, a people of whom I am a genetic part, had been sadistically eliminated by Germans, yet the people I felt relaxed and comfortable with were Germans. I hadn't expected this.

Travelling through the Baltic states and Poland put what post-war Germany has achieved into a more realistic perspective for me. And what that nation has achieved is simply this. Germany faced, acknowledged and accepted its past. When I meet an elderly German man, I cannot help but think, 'What did you do in the war? What did you know?' I have no such feelings for his children or grandchildren. In fact, it's the opposite. I trust and respect the old German's descendants because I know that, unlike many of those I have seen in

321

'new Europe', they are aware of their history. More than any other nation in Europe, they understand what depths humans are capable of sinking to.

We chatted at length about what parents end up doing for their grown children, about the pleasures of carrying your home on your back when travelling, and about the recent elections in Germany. She told me her friends questioned voting for Angela Merkell, for a woman chancellor. Her husband explained that Merkell lost votes because she is Protestant and from the East but then he went beyond immediate politics and made similar statements to those I had heard more than once since passing through northern Germany.

'We are a rich nation and we need to get our house in order,' he told me, '1989 would have been the ideal time to do it but we didn't do it very well. However, the infrastructure is now in place in the East. What is two per cent? We must tighten our belt. We have such short memories. German people have forgotten what poor means.'

'All Germans should come here to see what "poor" really means. Look at the devastation of 45 years of Communism,' his wife added.

When they asked where I was going, I explained there was a Lemko ethnologic museum around 15 kilometres away, near the Dukla Pass and a small 'Jewish Home Museum', the *'Muzealną Chatą Zydowską'*. She told me she thought it was an excellent idea and that she had done almost the same, taking her children to visit the farm near Szczecin where her grandparents and her mother had lived.

She didn't call it Stettin, but used the Polish name for the city from which Germans were expelled at the end of World War Two, when the Soviet Union annexed large parts of eastern Poland and 'gave' Poland over 100,000 square kilometres of German territory in compensation. Although the city of Stettin was west of the Oder-Neisse line that defined the new border between Poland and Germany, it was given to Poland because Stalin wanted Königsberg—now Kaliningrad—as a year-round port. When Stalin refused to let the Poles keep L'vov (now L'viv) he gave them Breslau (now Wroclaw). The defining purpose of the European Union was to end the need for any more of these kind of name changes.

That was a noble purpose, and it was supported both by the political elites and by the masses who had suffered so terribly in Europe's twentieth-century conflicts. This should still be the defining purpose of the European Union. I have no problem with expanding economic integration, not only with the countries I was travelling through but with those on their borders too, from the Ukraine down to Turkey, but I've got profound reservations about cultural, political and legal integration. That is an historical impossibility, a political fantasy.

I don't want to share a legal system with countries that culturally have no respect for law. I don't want to complete a similar tax return to other Europeans, knowing how in one culture—mine—honesty is generally assumed, while in other cultures, dishonesty is the norm. I don't want people who have been raised in a culture of smoke and secrecy making decisions that affect how I live.

Travelling through this region of Europe has

sharpened the realisation that I share my culture with only some parts of Europe—the Netherlands, Germany, Denmark, Sweden. The further I have travelled from these regions the more alien things have become.

I share a common humanity with the people I met, and more intimately, a common European heritage, but that doesn't mean we can become a political or cultural union. I don't think that I am alone in my beliefs. Everywhere I travelled, the people I met had misgivings about the direction the European Union is heading in.

* * *

Transit-man shared breakfast mushrooms with me and in return I gave him a tow to jump-start his old van. His alternator was on the blink—the Polish word for alternator, I learned, is '*alternator*'—and he'd been stranded there for three days, living off mushrooms and water from the stream.

MUSHROOM SOUP FOR BREAKFAST
Fry a mixed variety of finely chopped edible mushrooms in Polish butter and set them aside for the night.
Boil peeled potatoes in fresh water from a nearby stream.
Add salt and when the potatoes are completely softened, mash them into the water they were boiled in.
Add more butter and the fried mushrooms.
Drink, steaming hot, from enamel mugs.

I arrived at the Lemko Ethnologic and Jewish

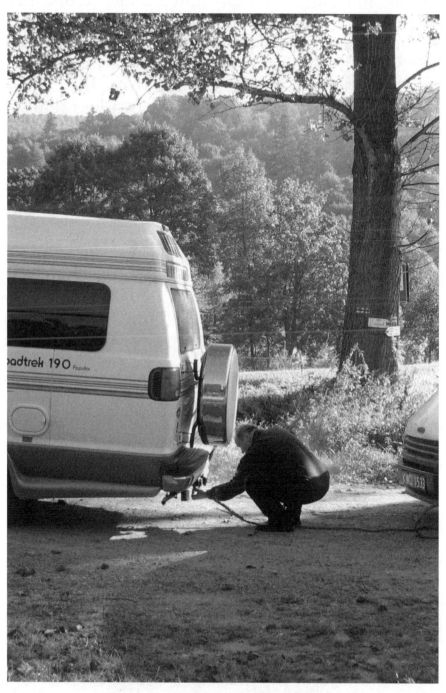

An early-morning tow near the border with Slovakia

Home museums at 8.30 a.m., long before they were due to open, so I just wandered around outside them, looking through the curtained windows. In the Jewish home each window had a candelabra in it—electric ones from Ikea. They only had seven candles on them, two less than on the nine-candled Jewish menorah but that harmless, even charming, mistake would go unnoticed by most who visited here.

Satisfied that I had seen at least one small acknowledgement by one man of the Jewish heritage of this part of Europe, I returned to the smooth-surfaced E road that curved through forested hills towards the nearby Slovak border. Truckers flashed their lights signalling me that police with a radar gun were hiding ahead, hoping to extract a final financial farewell from people leaving Poland.

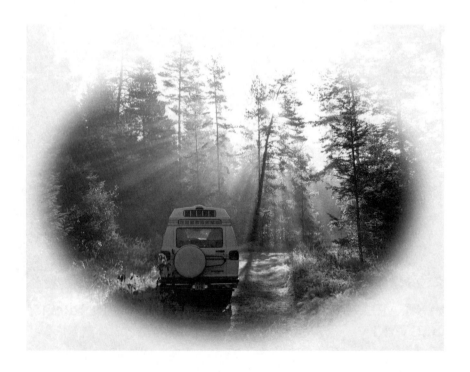

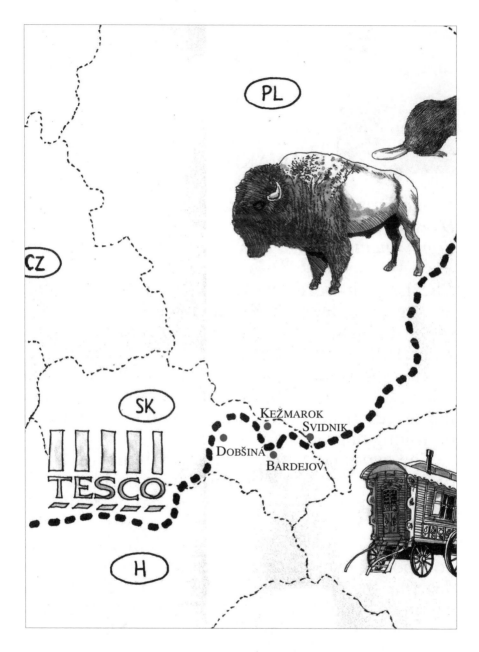

CHAPTER EIGHT

SLOVAKIA

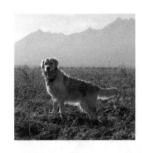

SLOVAKIA

People per square kilometre	*110*
Dogs per square kilometre	*17*
Roma unemployment rate	*90 per cent*

The English word 'gypsy' comes from the Greek for 'Egyptian': the Greeks thought the Roma came from the land of the Pharaohs, but they were several thousand miles short of the mark. Today we know that their ancestors came from the Indian subcontinent, and picked up plenty of cultural influences from other countries in the course of their long migration.

The gypsy language is akin to Hindi with traces of Slavonic and Greek thrown in, a heritage of its Indian origins and its lengthy sojourn in the Balkans. When I was at university, Django Reinhardt's 'gypsy music' was fashionable but it's now politically incorrect to use the word 'gypsy' to describe the people who played it, or the man from whom I bought a bucket of lingonberries in a Slovakian village. That Roma spoke Slovakian to me but Roma to his henna-haired mother. In this eastern region of Slovakia almost all the inhabitants in the desolate villages I drove through were Roma.

*   *   *

After waving goodbye to the Polish cops waiting patiently at the radar trap on their side of the border, I crossed through the Dukla Pass into the rump end of former Czechoslovakia, the easily forgotten Republic of Slovakia, an independent country since 1993. The Czechoslovak Republic came into existence in 1918 when the old Hapsburg Austro-Hungarian Empire collapsed. After the fall of Communism in 1989, Slovaks wanted to hyphenate the country's name and give their half more respect by calling it Czecho-Slovakia. While the majority of Czechoslovakians did not want to see their country broken up, self-interested politicians used the 'great hyphen debate' to further their own causes. Savvy Czech economists saw it was no loss to rid themselves of economically backward Slovakia, while the former Communist Party hacks in power in Slovakia realised it would be easier for them to retain personal power if the two countries separated.

And so it was. Bumping along a potholed highway, a kilometre past the Slovak frontier post where my documents had been scanned, checked, checked again, then checked again, I was stopped by six Slovakian guys in brown jackboots and green battle fatigues. One was waving a small red lollipop sign at me. As I pulled on to the shoulder of the road I was surrounded by four more thugs in black jackboots, black trousers and black jackets with *'Polizia'* embroidered on the right side, all carrying machine-guns. None were Roma. They all looked grim, like they were about to engage in TV wrestling.

329

I opened the driver's door and got out and so did Macy and on seeing my dog, the cops suddenly all backed off, like night crawlers when a light is shone on them. From behind them a giant of a guy strode forward, the dog handler. With his German shepherd barking venomously from inside his van, and with a face as darkly scowling as his black fatigues, he reassured his comrades.

'I'm a professional. I can handle blonde city bitches,' he told them in Slovak, or something like that. Macy cantered up to him and crotched him. From the flare of her nostrils I could tell he seldom changed his underwear. There wasn't a glimmer of amusement from the goon but his police colleagues tried hard to suppress their grins. I put her back in the camper.

'*Turistika?*' asked one of the men in green fatigues.

What do you say when you're asked such a stupid question? I'm a grey-haired guy with a foreign passport, travelling with a dog in a flash Canadian motorhome with British plates. Do I tell him his query is totally absurd?

'Yes, your majesty. I am a tourist,' I replied and I guessed right. He understood 'yes' and 'tourist'.

*   *   *

It was October and autumn had just touched this region. There were splashes of mustard on the forested hills. A mile beyond the spot check, I passed a Slovak police speed trap, then a billboard telling me it was only 91 kilometres to a culture I understood: a Tesco supermarket. There wasn't much traffic on this road although the Dukla Pass,

330

which, at only 500 metres above sea level, is the lowest crossing of the Carpathian Mountains and has been the chosen route of traders and armies for hundreds of years.

On the Great European Plain to the north, the successive acts of Europe's centuries-old civil war have taken place over a great swathe of land, opposing forces ebbing and flowing, but here in the centre of the hourglass, those battles were fiercely concentrated—especially in the last two centuries.

This was the route used by the Russian military to reach their battlefields with the Hungarians in the 1800s. It was the site of major battles in World War One and in World War Two where, in less than two months, almost 50,000 soldiers died and almost twice that many were maimed. Driving down from the Pass towards Svidnik I stopped in a valley, at a brook by a dirt road towards Kapišovà, to inspect one of the war memorials spattered throughout the area. On a concrete plinth was a German PZ-3 tank. On a higher plinth was a Soviet T-34 tank, positioned so that it was crashing down on the front of the German tank. The clash between East and West is still vivid here.

Svidnik is moderately interesting. Pedestrian crossing signs show a man wearing a fedora crossing the road. Old Skodas abound. The town itself was totally destroyed in World War Two and rebuilt by the Communists to conform to their starkly functional architectural principles. There is nothing of the vernacular, not a gabled roof in sight, but somehow the totality—the uniformity of angular concrete, sharp reflections, crisply defined lines—was impressive. I wasn't offended, as I had been by the Soviet buildings in the Baltic states and Poland.

Leaving town on a back road towards Bardejov, I passed an open-air war museum. Everywhere else I had visited in Eastern Europe all vestiges of the Soviet occupation had been removed, but here they were still proudly displayed. Jan Hana's *Memorial to the Red Army* has as a centrepiece a bronze statue of a Soviet sergeant, standing in front of a 37-metre high white-stone monument surmounted by a massive red star, surrounded by more impassioned white-stone statues and bas-reliefs of Red Army soldiers and grateful civilians. It's hagiography but it's wonderfully emotive hagiography. So too are the Red Army mortar launching vehicles, tanks, trucks and planes that litter the parklands, all with peeling red-painted stars on them.

No Western troops were involved in the grim battle of Dukla Pass, so it's not part of our war memory. My 'history' of World War Two has plucky little Britain holding out alone until the Americans, aided by the Canadians, join together and free Europe from German occupation. 'Our people' defeated Germany. But from the day I arrived in Estonia, another history has been apparent, a history that says that World War Two was not a battle between good and evil, but one that was fought between two loathsome evils: the Russian Communists and the German Nazis. 'We' didn't defeat Germany. Stalin's gruesome dictatorship, powerfully aided by us, did. Here, someone had just placed a wreath of fresh flowers at the feet of the Soviet sergeant.

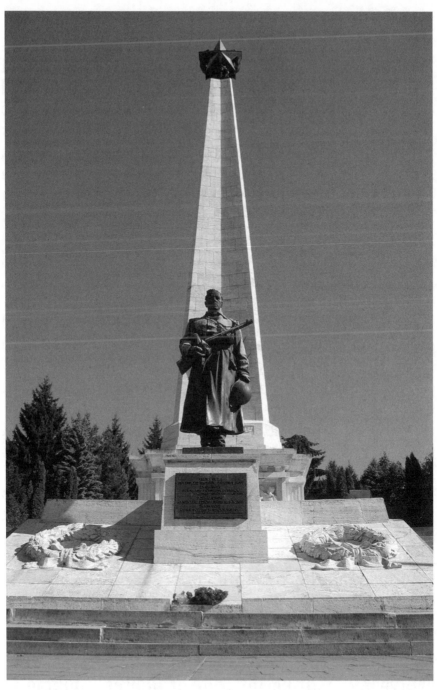

Jan Hana's *Memorial to the Red Army*, Svidnik

This remote region of Slovakia is called Carpatho-Ruthenia, a land that became part of Czechoslovakia only because of successful campaigning by Ruthenians who had emigrated to the United States. It's where the newspaper proprietor and crook Robert Maxwell came from. Across the road from the Red Army memorial is a Ruthenian ethnologic museum, another *skansen*.

Macy and I wandered briefly through the empty grounds, past buildings salvaged from villages in the region, but in the end I decided to press on and headed west, running alongside the Polish border, only a few kilometres away. The local government-issued rubbish bins by the roadside were faded galvanised metal, far more aesthetically attractive than the green or brown plastic bins that now desecrate British villages. The onion domes of Orthodox churches dominated the villages and initially all town signs were in the Roman alphabet with Cyrillic lettering underneath giving their Ruthenian names.

The style of homes in the villages I drove through was strikingly different to those across the border in Poland. There were rows of single storey homes all attached to each other, winding sinuously as the road meandered, and eventually developing into rows of two storey gable-roofed homes in the heart of the village then dropping back down one storey again as I left the village and returned to open pasture and fields. Roma were everywhere, sitting in front of houses, walking in groups, gathered in knots by trees. They were surprisingly dark skinned, as dark as Tamils. Many

334

of the boys had the quiffs of their gelled hair dyed blond. Some of the girls were strikingly beautiful, alluringly so—out of Bizet's *Carmen* or Puccini's *La Bohème*.

*   *   *

Bardejov is an exquisite medieval fortified town, immaculately preserved during the Soviet era. *Baedeker* said only of Bardejov: 'Bartfa, Ger. Bartfeld, a small and ancient town with 6100 inhabitants (one third Jews).' It was settled by Saxon weavers, and the cobbled, elongated, main square rises to the south, creating a beautiful panorama of pastel-coloured, steeply gabled, burghers' houses.

In front of the homes on each side of the wide square, are rectangular patches of grass, an attention to detail that was particularly admired by Macy and by the long-haired dachshund than followed her incessantly like a train caboose. Under a brilliant blue sky and in T-shirt weather I had a salami and cheese sandwich and a beer in one of the plastic tents in the square which had a sign outside reading, 'Irish Pub'. At the bottom of the square is the Bazilika, a Disneyesque, Gothic church, and immediately to the south of it a Renaissance town hall with a beautiful stone staircase.

There were no other tourists here, only a few people who looked as if they were locals. At the top of the square one of the stone and brick houses had been converted into an antique shop. I walked up its three stone steps, through two arched, Gothic, wooden doors and entered a stone-floored

335

corridor. A room opened to the left and it led to a smaller middle room with stairs to the next floor and then a large back room with a door to the backyard. I imagine this was the layout of all the houses in the square. All the rooms were filled with tat, stuff you find at car-boot sales—what the Swedes call *'loppis'*. The young academic-looking antique dealer enjoyed the opportunity to speak English. He explained that the EU was good for him because it meant more Western tourists, but Western tourists were not necessarily a 'good thing'.

'Why do the British drink so much?' he asked. 'The Swedes are the same. I had two Swedish girls living here last summer but they were more interested in vodka than anything else.'

I asked what happened to the Saxon inhabitants of Bardejov.

'The people here were Jews and German-speaking people from the Czech Republic. These people owned the sawmills and brickworks. Most business was owned by them. The Germans killed the Jews. Then after the war the Germans were transferred.'

That was an excellent euphemism. The Czechs and Slovaks 'transferred' millions of their German-speaking citizens in the years after World War Two. They rid their countries of them. Families may have lived here for 800 years but they were now 'others' to the victorious Czechs and Slovaks.

Remnants of their presence are the 'best buys' in antique shops, old books in German, left behind by those who were 'transferred'. I asked how large the Jewish population was and he explained that they had made up half of the entire population. I hadn't expected that and he told me that several of the old Jewish buildings including the synagogue are now undergoing restoration. I asked what had happened to the Soviet era collective farms and he explained that collective farmland is very cheap to buy but bureaucrats use red tape to make it almost impossible to use the land, 'Unless, of course you have lots of money to pay the bureaucrats to cut the red tape. The poor remain poor because they cannot afford these expenses. In the early days people thought we would become like Western Europe but now they realise that this is not so.'

I bought a heavy, old, cream-coloured linen bedspread from the antique dealer for Julia and some food from the local supermarket for Macy and me—rye bread, local salami, pasta, tomatoes, cheese-topped pastry, rolled herring in aspic and, of course, honey—then headed west, through rambling forested mountains, wildflower-filled meadows, past fortified castles on hills. An hour later the imposing range of the saw-toothed High Tatra Mountains suddenly came into view. Beyond the uninspiring town of Stara Ľubovna I found a campsite for the night.

RED STEW
Scald two large beefsteak tomatoes in boiling water, remove the skins and chop the tomatoes up.
Remove the seeds from four red peppers and chop them finely.
Chop up a red onion and fry in oil until it's golden, then move it to the side of the pan, add the chopped red peppers and gently fry them until they are soft.

Add the tomatoes, a squirt of tomato paste, ground pepper and salt and simmer for 20 minutes.
With the Tatra Mountains as a backdrop, eat with thick slices of freshly baked rye bread.

The following morning I crossed the Poprad river, traversed the flat plain of potato fields and on a secondary dirt road climbed into the foothills of the Tatras where I parked by a rapid stream— really a continuous waterfall. I had breakfast and took Macy for a walk upstream. There was a track of sorts that we stuck to through the woods, probably made by hunters. In the air was the musky smell of wild boar and Macy was in her element. This was a young mixed forest, mostly alders by the stream but also beech and spruce. I could hear thrushes. Macy worked the sides of the cascade, through honeysuckle and raspberry shrubs, taking care as she stepped from rock to rock, occasionally drinking from the running water. She joined me on the track and, tail high, lead the way until she stopped and investigated an odour from the path. It was a large animal scat. From its shape I knew it was a bear scat.

Slovakia is a refuge for Europe's greatest concentration of brown bears. There are so many bears that the country's carrying capacity is filling up, and now they wander across the borders, as far away as Germany. The population of around 800 is controlled by issuing licences to hunters to kill a varying number each year, while others are captured live and transported for relocation as far away as the French-Spanish Pyrenees.

I got a stick and poked around in the scat and it

seemed to be all fibrous vegetable material. At this time of year bears eat mostly fruit such as blueberries and lingonberries and mast such as beech nuts, acorns and pine nuts. Hunters intentionally set out food for wild boar and deer, and bears enjoy that too. They may be classified as carnivores but bears are not as efficient killers as wolves, pine martens, lynx and wildcats. Insects are a significant part of their diet and honey from wasp nests and bee-hives remains their preferred delicacy.

The scat was old and dried right through, but still I tethered Macy to me. At this time of year bears were fattening up for hibernation which would begin shortly, in November. I didn't want her to provoke a bear, or end up as dinner. We walked on but now my eyes were glued to the ground, searching for more bear scat.

Was the one Macy found deposited by a bear with a natural wariness of people or by one that has been conditioned to our presence because we provide a regular source of food? Was it a male or a female? If it was a female did she have young? Bear cubs are born in late winter, usually in pairs, weigh around the same as new-born beagle pups, (about 400 grams) then grow 50 times that size in their first year, thanks to their mother's milk. Cow's milk is around four per cent fat. Bear's milk, like seal's milk, is closer to 20 per cent fat.

Here, as elsewhere, wild carnivores such as bears and wolves polarise public opinion into seemingly irreconcilable camps: the conservationists, usually from cities, and the ruralists, usually farmers and hunters. How we handle wildlife is a social and political problem not

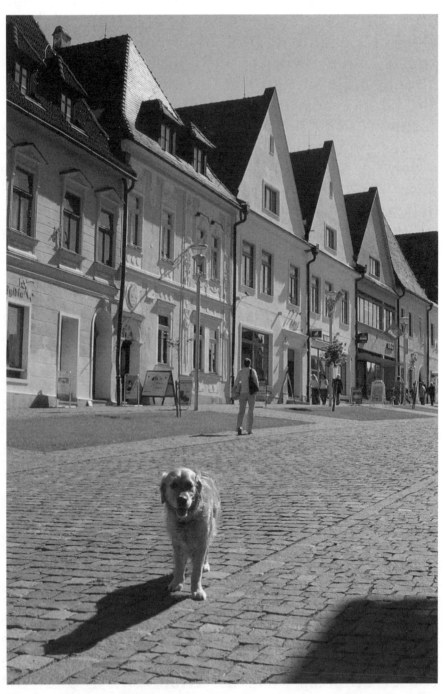

BURGHERS' HOUSES LINING THE STREETS OF
BARDEJOV

a scientific one. People on both sides of the argument pontificate according to their passions and perceptions.

Hunters and farmers exaggerate the numbers of wild carnivores and exaggerate the damage they inflict. They play upon our natural fear of predator animals because they know that we have a cultural limit for living with wild carnivores. Conservationists lie equally well, claiming species are in imminent danger of extinction while playing down the damage they cause to livestock or agricultural crops.

Dispassionate scientific fact might sound like the answer but what is 'fact' today might be proved wrong tomorrow. There is no answer to this problem because both sides are firmly and politically entrenched. Personally, I have no moral problem with biologically sound harvesting of surplus carnivores. If that means selling licences to bastards who get their testosterone kicks from killing noble animals, and using their blood money to enhance the environment for other wild animals, well, that's the way life is.

*   *   *

Back in the Poprad valley I was crossing the Spiš region, also settled by Saxons over 800 years ago. This was once a virtually independent region of the Hungarian kingdom, a mosaic of Slovaks, Germans, Hungarians, Poles, Ruthenians, Jews and Gypsies. Kežmarok is dominated by a gaudy, terracotta and cucumber-coloured Lutheran church, a weird combination of Moorish dome, stained-glass Stars of David, Renaissance tower

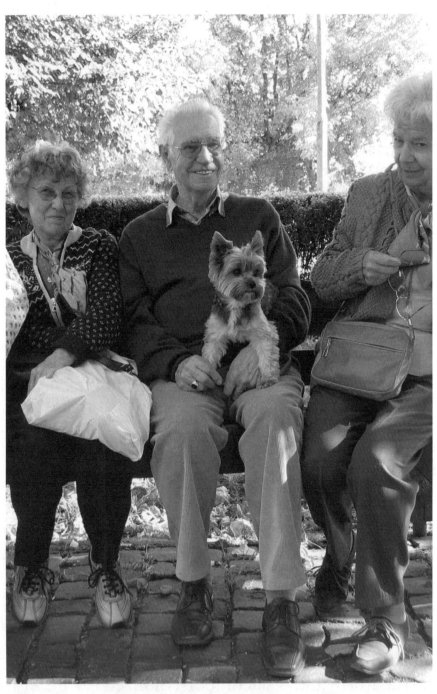

Locals with their coiffed and combed
Yorkshire terrier in Kežmarok

and defensive buttresses. Locals exercised their coiffed and combed Yorkshire terriers in the surrounding park.

In Kežmarok a sparkly, smiling girl stuck out a thumb for a hitch when she saw the Roadtrek. I was at a traffic light so I signalled her to jump in and this led to a short discussion amongst the hitchhikers.

'What are we doing?' asked one. 'He's an old foreign fart. We're interested in hunky guys with cheekbones like ours, as high as the Tatras.'

Sparky wasn't going to be put off by such nonsense. She bounded, grinning, to the back passenger door and hopped in. Her three friends followed, then two more. The oldest student, around 20, with frosted blonde hair pulled back with a ribbon, a big gap between her upper teeth, Christian Dior sunglasses in her hair, gold hoop-earrings and necklace, a deep tan, and a coral coloured cotton V-neck sweater bagged the front seat. Sparky got the seat immediately behind her.

'Where are you from?' they asked in unison and in English. Looking in my rear-view mirror, I saw two Slovakian mice sitting on the bed and three more girls sitting in a row on the floor. Macy didn't know what to think but she had her head tickled by all of them.

Coral practised her English by asking where I had been in Slovakia and where I was going. Halfway to Poprad she pointed to where she wanted to be let off. Sparky instantly stepped over Macy and bagged the front seat. She smiled endearingly and unendingly. The Spiš region of Slovakia is not exactly the cutting edge of cool and I, for a moment, was the most exciting event in this back of beyond since autumn term began.

Sparky radiated charm, while the mice sat meek and quiet.

'I love London,' she said, her knees tucked tightly under her chin.

I asked her when she had visited and she told me she hadn't, not yet, but she hoped to one day. In Poprad at an intersection surrounded by grey concrete high-rise Soviet era apartment towers. I dropped the academy students off and headed for the hilltop town of Levoča.

When I arrived in Levoča the town looked closed. I easily parked in the main square surrounded by terracotta and pastel-coloured, graffito'd burghers' houses and walked, first the square itself, then the surrounding grid of back streets, all within the ancient fortified walls.

*   *   *

The centrepiece of the square is the sixteenth-century Old Town Hall, a squat, heavyweight blockbuster of columns, arches, pillars, arcades and, as everywhere in this region of Slovakia, extraordinarily high-stepped gables. All the buildings in the square were immaculately restored. This was once the most wealthy town in the region, a centre of trade in copper, leather, wax, fur, plums and wine. I stopped for a drink and pastry at one of the restaurants that had outdoor tables on the pavement and Macy was given a bowl of water.

The back streets, with their commanding views of the valley below, were still in protracted hibernation. Once the homes of successful Saxon

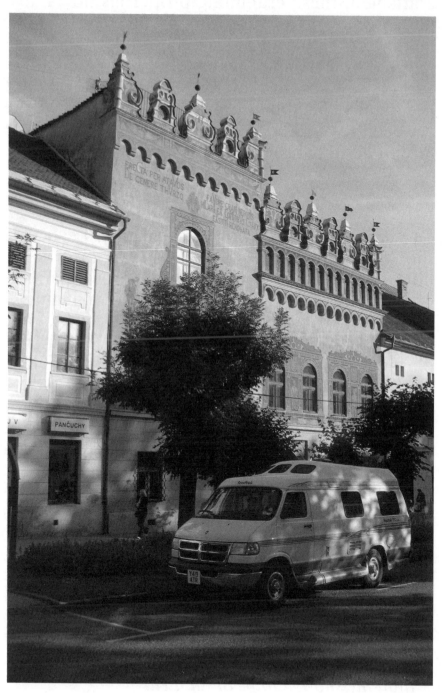

THE TOWN SQUARE IN LEVOČA

craftsmen, these crumbling properties now house poor Roma and Slovaks who, in the late-afternoon light were gathered in gaggling knots. Macy was taunted by a group of teenagers who barked at her and chased her on their bicycles but she retained her dignity. The buildings are elegant but have not yet been re-awakened by the kiss of tourism or the lure of homes abroad to Western Europeans.

*   *   *

Our campsite, three kilometres north of Levoča, in the woods by Levočská Dolina, was on a steep hill. There was a cascade of brown-painted, green-roofed bungalows that looked strikingly like ranks of oversized Lithuanian beehives, and surrounding them on three sides there was parking, with electricity, for motorhomes. There was only one other camper at the grounds.

The campsite German shepherd was wearing a muzzle when I checked in at the office, and the reason became obvious when we parked in our slot. Within seconds of Macy emerging from the Roadtrek the shepherd attacked, going for Macy's neck. I pulled the slavering dog off and held her until the campsite gardener arrived, put her on a leash and marched her indoors where she remained for the rest of our stay.

SPICY SLOVAKIAN SUPPER
Slice and dice spicy, dried, rough Bardejov pork sausage and toss gently in a buttered frying pan until the snowy lumps of fat melt.
Slice and dice half a large onion, add it to the sausage in the pan and fry until golden. Set both

aside.

Slice a microwaved potato and fry it in the pan until the slices take on some colour, then add the fried sausage and onion.

Pour in two eggs that you have blended with a fork and cook until the combination sets.

Sprinkle with chopped Polish chives, place a shotgun on your knees to see off Slovakian shepherd dogs and eat quickly before the dusk mosquitoes drive you crazy.

The cold night air drove the mosquitoes away but in the warm dawn sunshine they returned. I found an old logging trail up into the hills and climbed the deeply wooded forest. It was hard work. I got puffed out and stopped intermittently but Macy was in high gear, disappearing up over the steep bank at the edge of the track and into the woods, obviously scent trailing. On a particularly arduous section of the trail I saw why.

Wild boar had been rooting and from the freshness of the overturned soil I could tell they had been there very recently—no more than a few hours ago. I inhaled lightly and now I too could smell them. Mace crashed through the underbrush and with resignation I let her. In her surge of predatory excitement there was no way I'd be able to get her to return until she was in sight of me.

Within 10 minutes she was back, bristling with excitement. She jumped down from the height of the surrounding woods on to the trail but didn't realise there was a deep rain rut hidden under the undergrowth. Her right foreleg took the full weight of the unexpected drop and she emerged holding it up.

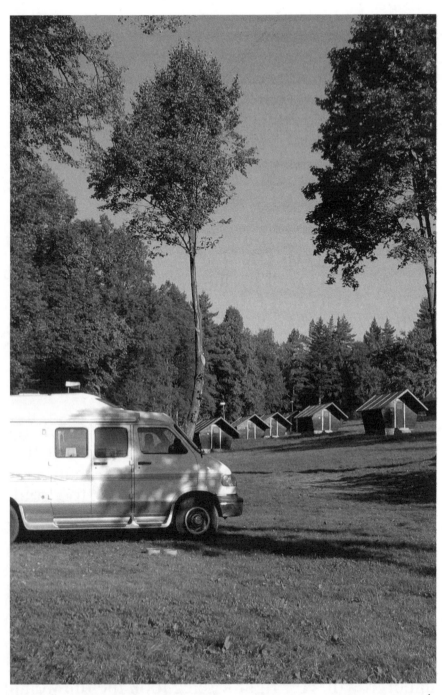

Our campsite in the woods by Levočská Dolina

She couldn't bear weight on it and cried out gently when I touched it. I sat her down and let her panting excitement diminish then carefully examined the limb from the toes to the shoulder. There were no breaks but great discomfort to the top of the limb. I massaged the region and after 10 minutes she put the leg down. After another 10 minutes of rubbing, she hobbled and bore some of her weight on it. With her lead on, we slowly walked back down to the campsite, had breakfast and were gone by 8.30 a.m.

*   *   *

I headed south to the 'Slovenkský Raj National Park' or the 'Slovakian Paradise National Park'. Communication lines and roads in Slovakia run east and west. To go from north to south involves undertaking unending hairpin turns over mountainous roads. This is fine in a car, but in a heavy motorhome with an injured dog, driving took concentration. The guard rails along the roads had massive dents in them. Some sections had been broken clean through and beyond were precipitous drops to oblivion. Tailgating Tatra logging trucks, including one with an incongruous American confederate flag on its grille, tried to intimidate me to drive faster but with my ears popping and the inclines and declines at 12 per cent, I remained resolute.

Villages straddled the road in the deep valleys between the hills and in those villages, sitting on fences, walking in groups, or running to the road to display buckets of berries to passing vehicles, were more Roma. I stopped to see what they had

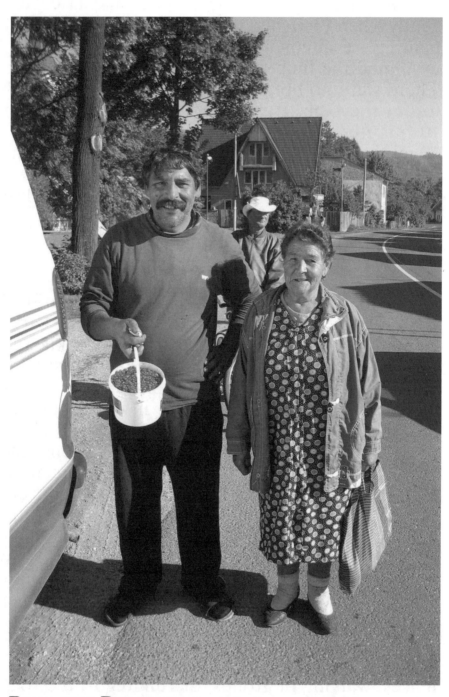

ROADSIDE ROMA PEDDLING THEIR WARES

and how much they wanted for the berries.

No one knows exactly how many Roma live in Slovakia. They constitute probably around five per cent of the total, a community living on the social periphery of the predominant Slovak population, yet in the villages I had driven through since arriving from eastern Poland they appeared to be in the majority.

During World War Two the Germans carried out mass killings of Roma but they were not as efficient killing them as they were killing Jews. There are around 2000 Jews left in Slovakia, all speaking Slovakian and between 250,000 and 400,000 Roma most of whom speak the Slovak Carpathian Romany language as well as Slovakian in an eastern Slovak dialect.

Throughout their entire history in Slovakia, their language was only spoken, never used in books, newspapers or other publications. It was only after the numerous local Romany dialects were codified and standardised that the Romany language began to appear in children's stories, poems and memoirs in the 1990s.

Roma have their own languages, their own culture and an intensely problematic future. Without the strong influence of a unifying religion, or an ancestral homeland to aspire to return to, or a history that rewards education, social or cultural development, the Romany remain steeped in a pit of inferiority. They are certainly treated as second-class citizens here, the ultimate 'others'.

*   *   *

In the heart of the Slovenský Raj, amongst the

steep limestone hills and deep, shady ravines I descended through the spruce forest to Dedinský, and a large open reservoir where men in rowboats were fishing. We walked by a stream and I picked some water mint. A billboard by the highway told me microwaves were on sale at Tesco for 1499 korunas (£22.50).

Beyond the logging village of Dobšiná I stopped by a field of dried sunflowers for lunch and below a tree filled with squawking magpies, I shared tomatoes, cheese, sausage, rye bread and raspberries with Macy. Here in south-eastern Slovakia the town signs were now both in Slovak and Hungarian. Hungarians make up the largest minority group in Slovakia. Just before the border crossing into Hungary I passed two goats tied to a tree, headbutting each other.

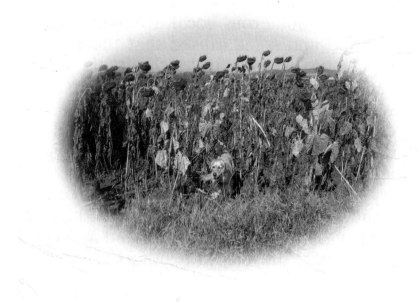

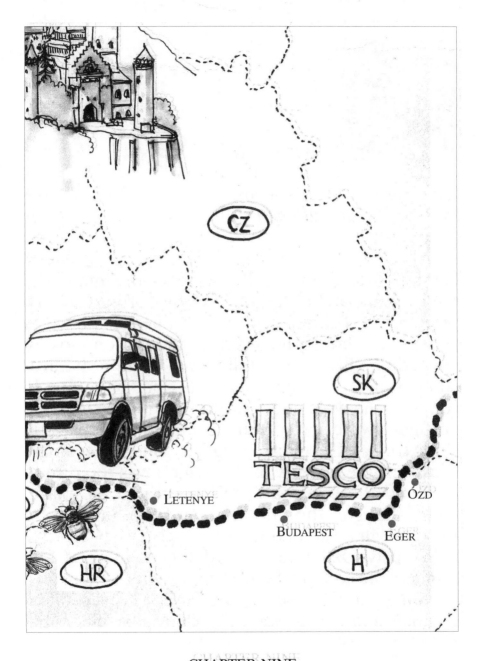

CHAPTER NINE

HUNGARY

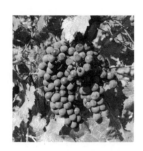

HUNGARY

People per square kilometre	*108*
Dogs per square kilometre	*20*
Grapes stolen	*3 kilos*

Peter Kertész, my family dentist—the man who removed the painfully infected tusk from Carl the elephant at Tallinn Zoo in Estonia—was born in Hungary, although he has lived in London most of his adult life. He tells me that whatever Hungarians do, they want to be best at. In Hungary the welcome signs to the villages I passed through were at their ecumenical best, in Hungarian, German, English and Slovakian. However, the poverty in this region was too dire to hide and there was a desolate aura to the place, even though the natural surroundings were abundant in autumn bounty.

In dusty Ózd I turned off the main road and climbed the hills to Szilvásvárad where there is a breeding centre for Lipizzaner horses. The original stud is further west, in Lipica, Slovenia, where I would visit in a few days' time. The Hungarian stud was created over 200 years ago to save the Lipizzaners in Lipica from Napoleon's troops. When Yugoslavia imploded in the 1990s, it was the Austrians' turn to carry out the rescue mission of the Lipizzaners from Slovenia.

Lipizzaners are dark-coated at birth but by six years of age are grey or white. They are relatively short legged and long backed, with thick necks and muscular thighs that give them a powerful presence. I'm deeply allergic to them, which is an embarrassing admission for a vet. At the Spanish Riding School in Vienna, where they bow and pirouette indoors under immense chandeliers, my chest seizes up whenever I watch them and I have to rush outside to catch my breath.

I descended, along the old road, twisting and turning through the Bükk Hills, to Eger, a bustling baroque town with a massive Tesco on the outskirts, and parked in front of a mustard-coloured Franciscan church on Kossuth Street before going for a stroll. I stopped not far from the ramparts to Eger Castle for some sickly sweet marzipan pastry and a decent coffee. Nearby in the sunlit square, a jazz quartet was playing Erroll Garner's 'Misty'. Mace finished the marzipan pastry and proceeded, on a sugar high, through the narrow streets to the castle itself. We backtracked to the striking, 40-metre high minaret, all that remains of the Turkish occupation of this region, then crossed the narrow, fast-flowing River Eger once more and wandered through the football-pitch sized Dobó István Square where there is a sumptuously impressive twin-towered baroque church.

Back at the Roadtrek, Macy was, as ever, reluctant to get back in and she dithered by the door. An elderly 'Viennese' woman of the sort that populated Louis' Patisserie in Hampstead in the early 1970s, spoke to me, in Hungarian. She was dressed in a brown, grey and green tweed suit with her jacket belted at the waist, had a small, round, rimmed, felt hat on her head, and was carrying a brown handbag and off-white gloves. She spoke with a smile in her eyes and in her voice, I'm sure about Macy's reluctance to get in the camper.

Macy finally got in the vehicle and I fished out my map to plan the next stage of my route. A minute later the woman returned and, I think, asked if she could see Macy again. My dog willingly jumped back down on to the pavement and the woman tentatively touched Macy on her back, then on her head, then patted her, then petted her, then stroked her. I stood mute, and was desperately sad that I couldn't understand a single word she was saying. How odd it is that a seemingly innocuous encounter can become a seminal moment. I'd met many other people in the last month who I couldn't converse with, but somehow this event was different. I wanted to know this woman, to have a coffee with her, to listen to her story, to tell her what Macy and I had been doing. Suddenly, my travels raced away from me. I'd had enough of rural peasantry, of rustic poverty. I'd had my fill of Europe's alien and painful past. This dignified, prim, urbane, urban 'elderly aunty' was someone I wanted to know yet I couldn't communicate with. I'd had enough of being on my own and wanted to return to the familiar. Back in the Roadtrek, after she had gone, I telephoned Julia and asked if she could meet me in Venice. Her immediate, 'Yes! Yes! Yes!' cheered me up though I didn't, as she asked me, kiss Macy for her. Julia kisses Macy a lot.

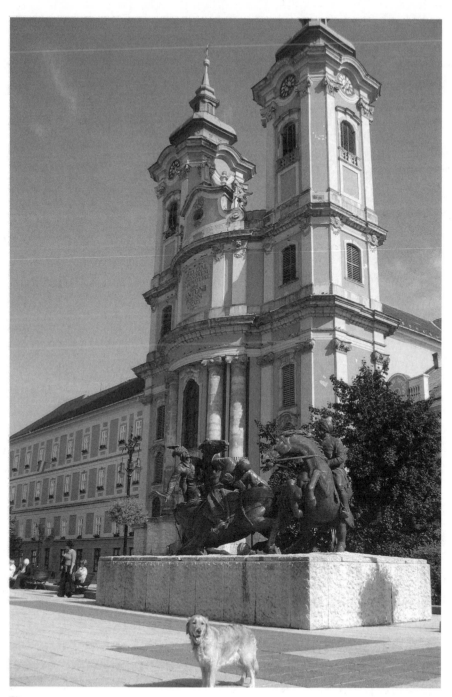

EGER, A BUSTLING BAROQUE TOWN

South of Eger I passed fields of just-harvested watermelons, guarded by sleeping tan-coloured mastiff dogs, and on the hills descending to the great Hungarian plains I stopped and picked—well, I stole—three kilos of deepest blue-coloured Kékfrankos grapes.

Eger's wealth was based on these grapes and they're still grown on the horseshoe of hills surrounding the town. In Germany the same grape is called the 'Limberger' although American growers in the State of Washington's Columbia River Valley changed that name to 'Lemberger'. They didn't want to produce a wine that was mistaken for smelly cheese. (Similarly, American dog breeders changed the name of the Hungarian guarding breed, the Komondor to the 'Kommander' but that's only because they thought the Hungarians got the original spelling wrong.)

The same late-ripening grape is grown in Austria, where it is the 'Blaufrankisch', but here in Hungary it is 'Egri Bikavér', the major variety for producing the local, full and fruity red wine with the nightmare name of Bull's Blood.

I had a choice between the old Highway 3 to Budapest or the brand-new E71 and Macy thanked me and slipped into a deep peaceful sleep when I chose the latter. There were no Trabants or old Skodas on this road over the pancake plain, only BMW 7s, Audi 8s and Mercedes tanks—'muscle' cars, often with Romanian, Bulgarian and Greek licence plates.

The next time you throw a coin in the fountain in the Piazza Navona in Rome, pause to look at Bernini's Fountain of Four Rivers: Africa's Nile, Asia's Ganges, South America's Plate and Europe's Danube. The Plate seems an odd choice for the Americas but the Danube is the right river to represent Europe south of the Great European Plain. It defines this region of Mitteleuropa.

From the depths of the Black Forest, it flows as the 'Donau', past Ulm and Regensburg in Germany, Linz and Vienna in Austria, as the 'Dunaj' through Bratislava in Slovakia, on to where I now was, stuck in rush-hour traffic, fighting TIRs on a bridge over the mighty 'Duna' river in Budapest, a river that my dentist Peter boated on as a small boy.

I'd been to Budapest several times previously, in the mid-1970s with Julia during the Soviet era, when Hungary was 'the happiest wing in the prison' and then again in 1990, less than a year after the orderly collapse of the People's Republic of Hungary and its succession by the Republic of Hungary, to lecture at the Budapest veterinary school. In 1991, when I returned, accompanied by my daughter Tamara, to give another series of lectures at the local veterinary school, it was Tamara who noticed the proud sign outside a restaurant where we ate, 'Established in 1989'.

In the twentieth century Hungary consistently chose the losing side. Germanised in its culture, educational system and administration, and tied to Austria and Germany by treaties, it fought on the side of the Central Powers in World War One and was dragged to defeat. The new states of Czechoslovakia, Romania and Yugoslavia, established at the Paris Peace Conference in 1920, were created from what had been Hungarian soil. Hungary lost over 60 per cent of its territory, and millions of its Hungarian-speaking population.

My visit in 1990 was my first chance to talk at length to people who until the previous year, had been inaccessible behind the Iron Curtain. A veterinary epidemiologist, on staff at the vet school, where students now could choose to study in Hungarian, German or English, had been one of the East Germans who realised in May 1989 that they could bypass the wall that divided East and West Germany and cross to the West through Hungary, where the barriers, barbed wire and minefields along its border with Austria had just been removed.

I asked what his first impression of Vienna was and he told me that what he saw was simply incomprehensible to him. 'The shops were filled with goods, yet nobody was shopping,' he explained. 'I could not understand how there could be so many goods, so much choice and no one was buying them. I had to sit down and reorganise my mind.'

The Hungarian veterinarians I had dinner with in 1990 spoke longingly of 'Greater Hungary', of reclaiming their Hungarian-speaking populations in Slovakia, Slovenia, Croatia, Serbia but especially in Romania. Their talk was sinister. Frightening. Not unlike what Slobodan Milosevic was saying about Greater Serbia. There is still an accident waiting to happen in this region of Europe.

＊　　　＊　　　＊

I knew Peter was Hungarian-born but didn't know his story until 1995, when he and I were in Nimfeon in the Greek hills by the Macedonian border. Peter was operating on six rescued dancing bears who were suffering chronic pain from multiple tooth root abscesses. He told me that although he had lived in London from the age of 13, and although he still felt thoroughly Hungarian, he was, officially, born Swedish. His birth certificate states that his mother was a Swedish national.

Budapest was in the grip of an incomprehensible evil in the summer of 1944, when Peter's short-sighted mother tripped over a pile of corpses on a street in Buda and went into premature labour. Accompanied by her own mother, she made her way to the nearby Janos Sanatorium but, as Jews—they were wearing obligatory yellow Stars of David—they were told to go away as 'Jews were not allowed to have children'. Peter's grandmother told his mother they should return to the Swedish House, where they lived, and when the sanatorium staff heard those words they asked to see Peter's mother's documents. She had a Swedish passport. The staff at the sanatorium delivered the baby.

Peter's Hungarian mother and grandmother had been given Swedish nationality documents by the Swedish diplomat Raoul Wallenberg. Peter's father hadn't. It was too late for him. He had already been picked up by the Gestapo and put to work in a slave labour camp. After Peter's birth, and back at the immensely crowded Swedish House, where

361

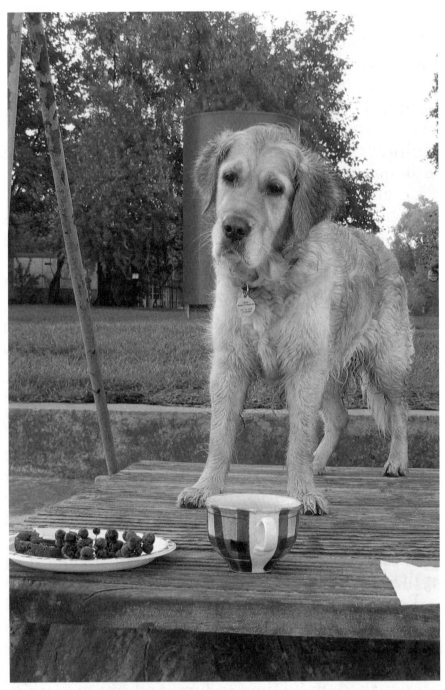

LAKESIDE BREAKFAST AT KODÁLY ZOLTÁN UTCA

their safety was assured because of their Swedish paperwork, Peter's mother had a photo taken of her new son and enclosed it in a letter she sent to her imprisoned husband. Weeks later it was returned, unopened. Peter has that letter.

'The Hungarians made sure they were always the best,' Peter told me, 'the best Nazis, the best anti-Semites, the best Communists.' Peter's father survived both the slave labour camp and a Gestapo prison and when the war ended, the Kertész family—Kertész is Hungarian for 'gardener'— were able to return to a semblance of normal life in a totalitarian state, living in a flat on Dohány utca, or 'Tobacco street', in English.

Before World War Two, Jews had created both ideas and wealth in Hungary, but parochial Hungarian nationalism, in ascendancy ever since the dissolution of the Austro-Hungarian Empire, had not been tempered by the war, nor even by the horrors of the industrial extermination of Hungary's Jewish and gypsy citizens.

In post-war Hungary, non-Magyars who asserted their own identity were still considered subversive. When Peter first went to kindergarten in Budapest in the late 1940s, he remembers his mother telling him to say he was Protestant, though he had no idea what that meant. Before the war, many Hungarian Jews had left, mostly for Britain or the United States, like the conductors Istvan Kertész and Sir George Solti; the photographers Andre Kertész and Robert Capa; the director of *Casablanca*, Michael Curtiz (Mihaly Kertész); the producer of *The Third Man*, Sir Alexander Korda; the screenwriter of Alfred Hitchcock's *49th Parallel*, Emeric Pressburger;

nuclear scientists Leó Szilárd and Edward Teller. So did Peter's Uncle Endre, a violinist who was a soloist with the Halle Orchestra in Manchester and who now lives in Malmö, Sweden. Other Hungarian Jewish families stayed and, as with Peter's family, some members survived. Imre Kertész, the novelist and recent recipient of the Nobel Prize for Literature, is one of them.

Peter's childhood in Hungary was an entirely urban one but his father had a rowing boat with a small outboard motor and they would go boating on the mighty Danube, until inevitably the motor failed each time and they needed rescuing. Uncle Endre kept in touch but the Kertész family remained locked in Hungary without passports.

In 1957, after the Hungarian revolution of October 1956, life became almost intolerable, but Peter's father was able to meet people who could make things happen and was able to exchange his flat on Dohány utca with a secret service policeman, in return for travel documents allowing his family to take a trip to nearby Vienna. Peter's father took his stamp collection with them and sold the stamps in Vienna for £500. Later, when he tried to deposit the notes in a London bank, he learned they were German forgeries from the Second World War. The family was penniless.

In England Uncle Endre ensured they had housing and arranged for Peter to study at an English boarding school. I met Uncle Endre, when he was in his nineties, and he had travelled to London to be with his nephew when Peter was the first dentist to become an Honorary Associate of the Royal College of Veterinary Surgeons for his contributions to animal welfare.

Raoul Wallenberg was seized by the Russians and disappeared for ever into the Soviet gulag. Peter is one of those who are known as 'Wallenberg's children', those who live because Wallenberg provided the protection of Swedish nationality. There is a Raoul Wallenberg Memorial Garden on Wesselényi utca in Budapest, less than 200 metres from where Peter lived and, in one of those apposite coincidences, on Great Cumberland Place, near Marble Arch in London, less than 300 metres from where Peter spends his working life.

*   *   *

All the campsites at Lake Balaton were closed for the season, so I camped at the end of Kodály Zoltán utca, by the 'beach' and sat on a dock watching the twinkle of lights from across the lake and, as swans glided by and gulls argued, shared a salami sandwich with Macy.

After Peter's father had brought his family here for a two-day holiday in the late 1940s, he was arrested and imprisoned for two days. The authorities wanted to know where he got the money for the holiday. The weather was now warmer, climbing into the mid-20s during the day, and the following morning we walked the 'beach'—in reality an unending grass-covered promenade along the milky, lime-green waters of the shallow lake.

During the summer season it is littered with Hungarians visiting the nearest thing to a seaside in this landlocked country. Lake Balaton is the largest lake in Europe outside Sweden, almost

LAKE BALATON, THE LARGEST LAKE IN CENTRAL
EUROPE

80 kilometres long and mostly 10 to 14 kilometres wide. In October, there were only dog walkers. We were yapped at by chihuahuas and, while I had breakfast on a dock and caught up on my writing, Macy played with a Hungarian sheepdog—a turbulent *'puli'* with a long, dreadlocked coat.

*   *   *

A new motorway from Budapest to Zagreb was nearing completion, but I avoided the already opened sections and, heading towards Slovenia, took the old road along the southern shore of the lake—a road lined with evening primroses on the verges and commercial apple orchards in the surrounding fields. The laden trees were pruned low for hand harvesting. A soft morning light, almost like a heat haze, shrouded the countryside.

I drove through the Kis-Balaton marshes at the southern end of the lake, a natural filter for water from the River Zala entering Balaton, drained by the Communist authorities, and now being restored in an attempt to improve the health of the lake. After miles of reclaimed farmland, now reverting back to marsh, I emerged from the flats, up a small incline into farmed land, dotted with neat villages, through fields of sunflowers being harvested and dried corn sitting in cribs.

Although it was autumn, fluorescent red poppies lined the fresh tarmac on to a brand new section of empty motorway. Magpies took off and landed on the empty road *en masse* and along the verges thousands of new saplings had been planted, sometimes four to six deep, occasionally even 10 to 15 trees deep. Beyond were vineyards and fields of drying corn. The road gently curved, rose and fell then ascended once more, up over a series of rolling hills towards Slovenia.

The motorway leads to Croatia and Zagreb, but I turned off and headed north to cross into Slovenia. Soon there will be a motorway here too: it's already being built. The old road still gives you a feel for the landscape, meandering through a series of nondescript villages. I passed a Trabant parked under a row of trees on the old road. A family with young children was harvesting fallen chestnuts. At a used-car lot in Letenye, a loose Caucasian Owtcharka was on security patrol. Mourning doves sat sunning themselves on the highway, fluttered up at my approach, and settled back down once I had passed. I stopped in a deeply wooded ravine and went walking in the spongy damp forest, surrounded by twittering finches popping from branch to branch in the saplings. There was mistletoe in the trees and a long line of parked transport trucks as I reached the border with Slovenia.

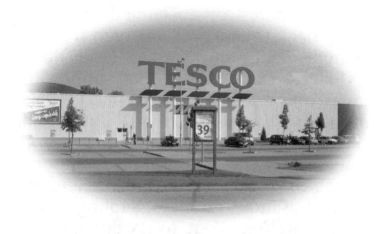

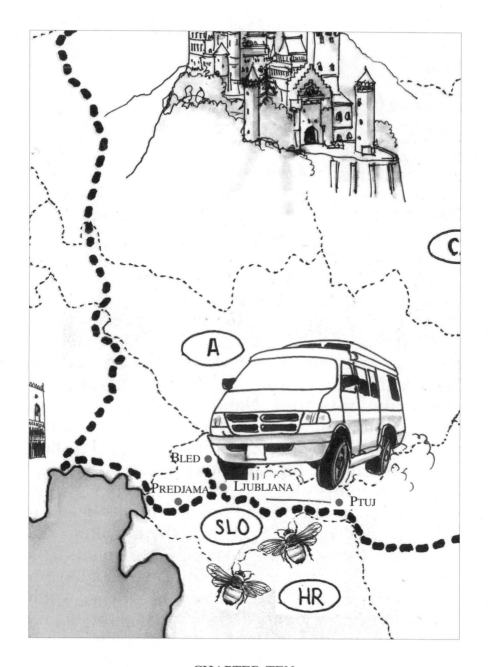

CHAPTER TEN

SLOVENIA

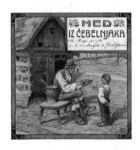

SLOVENIA

People per square kilometre	*100*
Dogs per square kilometre	*10*
Slovenians per beehive	*12*

A brief history of a curious country. There's a local breed of dog called the Illyrian shepherd, named after 'Illyria', or what is now Slovenia and Croatia. 'Illyria' was an ephemeral creation of the Napoleonic era. During the French occupation of this region of Europe, Napoleon lifted the ban on the Slovenian language and during that temporary separation of the country from Austrian Hapsburg rule a nationalist 'Illyrian' movement began.

By the mid-1800s the movement had split in two. Slovenian and Croatian aspirations began to diverge. Slovenians began to cultivate their own language, intentionally making it distinct from Croatian. The Croatians aligned their language to the neighbouring Serbians. Eventually it would become virtually identical to Serbian, although the former was written in Latin script, and the latter in Cyrillic. This proved to be good for me, because my dog and cat books now get translated into three languages, Slovenian, Croatian and Serbian.

In 1929, the 'Kingdom of Serbs, Croats and Slovenes' became the Kingdom of Yugoslavia and although it was the Slovenians and Croatians who initiated joining with the Serbians, they eventually came to resent the Serbian's dominance of the union.

In 1964 I visited the Federal People's Republic of Yugoslavia, driving up from Greece, through Macedonia, Serbia, Croatia and Slovenia and on to Italy. The exchange rate was 750 dinars to the American dollar, a litre of petrol cost 90 dinars or 15 cents and a luxury room the size of a ballroom at Belgrade's Grand Hotel Moscow cost 3600 dinars. A meal of smoked meats, *shashlik*, rice, tomato and onion salad, pasty, wine and cognac was 1600 dinars.

In Belgrade I'd visited the Fourth of July Museum, the Twenty-fifth of May Museum, the Museum of the First Serbian Uprising, the Military Museum of the Yugoslav People's Army, the Museum of the Underground Party Press. And you know, until I reread my diary from that trip I'd forgotten all about that.

In the countryside oxen and donkeys were still common modes of transport and people looked unkempt and poorly dressed, but in Belgrade I'd met Nena, Anna and Illya and I'd written that they were 'smartly dressed, well-groomed and good-looking'. In the evenings everyone walked, talked and, according to what I wrote, 'hummed'!

Nena spoke self-taught English and told me she hated Yugoslavia. She hated the language, the people, the fact she couldn't do what she wanted, and what she wanted was to visit the West, to visit Germany, France and America. She asked me what I thought of her country and I told her that people were friendly and looked happy, much like in other countries I'd visited. She told me it would probably be difficult for me to understand but the people only *looked* happy. Inside they were not. She said it was a charade. There was no individuality, no freedom to tell others your thoughts, no right to determine your own life. I listened and I didn't. Nena wanted to discuss politics. I wanted to get her in my sleeping bag.

* * *

In the flatlands of north-eastern Slovenia, as in Hungary, there were fields of squash, all slashed open with their seeds removed and their flesh left to rot. Driving towards Ptuj I stroked Macy and felt another tick on her chest. I'd removed so many I thought I'd remove this one while driving, and without looking, pinched and rotated it at its root. Macy winced and pulled away. I'd tried to remove her right front teat!

The village homes were pristine, geranium bedecked, freshly painted, with neat, manicured lawns. Some homes had displays of dried corn and squashes at their front doors. Beside the highway was a pathway for tractors and horse-drawn vehicles.

It was Saturday afternoon but compact, medieval Ptuj was empty. I parked near the small town square and in warm, bright sunshine we walked the narrow cobbled streets, past ancient homes, all furnished with Renaissance stone portals and all covered by sun-bleached, cracked stucco work and peeling paint that reminded me of the alleyways of Venice. The Old Irish Pub on narrow, cobbled Murkova ulica was enticing but it was in the shade so I returned to the Europa café in the town square for a coffee and asked for a bowl of water for Macy.

'You are English,' the young man at an adjacent table commented. 'Nice dog. Do you know the cross of St. George is also the coat of arms of this town?' and he grinned mischievously.

Jan and his two friends were visiting local vineyards. I'd ordered a '*krofi*', sort of a deep fried solid round doughnut but Jan suggested I have '*gibanica*', a cheese-filled strudel, which I tried and it was delicious. Macy enjoyed the *krofi* more than I did, but judged it second rate compared to the Tim Horton and Krispy Kreme doughnuts she'd lived on in Canada and the United States.

Everywhere I travelled in the new EU I encountered mixed feelings about membership but there was no hesitation on the part of Jan and his friends when I asked them about it.

'The EU, it is good for us,' he told me. 'Slovenia was not true part of Balkans. In EU we not go back to Balkans. We have small country mentality. It is no problem having two capitals. Belgrade was our other capital. Vienna was our other capital. Now Brussels is our other capital. This is no problem for us. It is our history to have two capitals.'

GIBANICA
Blend three small eggs into 500g of cottage cheese.
Add a cup of creamy milk, a quarter cup of sunflower oil and a large pinch of salt, then beat thoroughly until all are well-blended.
If you like, poppy seeds, walnuts and apple can

373

be added before blending.
Place a plain layer of filo pastry on a greased cooking pan and cover with a layer of the cheese batter.
Dip a thin layer of filo pastry in the batter and lay on top of the first.
Repeat with several more layers of dipped batter, topping the pile with a couple of layers of undipped filo pastry, making sure the top layer covers the sides and the ends of the pile.
Spoon some remaining batter on top, dot with pieces of butter and wash the top with milk.
Cook in the oven at around 170°C for 40 minutes.
If at first you don't succeed, modify the recipe and try again. When it works it's delicious.

I joined the A1 motorway towards Ljubljana, a toll road where I had the choice of paying in local currency or in euros. This choice was available everywhere I went in Slovenia. It was a beautiful drive, the most alluring of any I made on this trip. Afternoon light shone on small vineyards and their adjacent homes, on fields of hops, on church spires standing to attention on the heights of land. The road cut through mountains and bridged gorges and valleys. Tunnels were 700 metres long, then 1600 metres long, then 2800 metres in length, all followed by equally long viaducts. In the distance, mountain ranges shimmered in shades of mauve, blue and grey, melding into the western skyline.

Modern Slovenia's image makers have a problem. How do you capture the tourist market? How do you create a unique national identity when your image is wholly intertwined with other

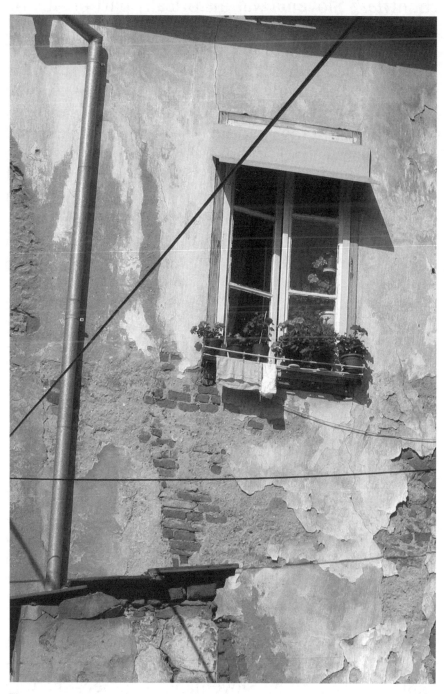

BACK STREET WINDOW IN PTUJ

countries? Slovenia was historically part of Austria and, for a brief interlude in the twentieth century, part of the 'Union of Southern Slavs' or Yugoslavia. The deepest roots of its identity remain stubbornly Austrian though—Alpine Austrian—and when I see the country's tourist material, enticing people to visit its lakes and mountains, I find it hard to see the difference between these mountains of Slovenia and those of Austria, just across the border. But I have a cunning way to distinguish the two cultures.

There is something truly unique about this small country, a quirk that instantly differentiates Slovenians from all its neighbours. Slovenians love bees: they are addicted to bee-keeping. They are downright nationalistic when it comes to their indigenous Slovenian bee. There are 8000 bee-keepers and 165,000 beehives in a tiny country with a population less than that of Toronto or Sidney.

*   *   *

Before I left on my travels I asked the vet I share the clinic with, Veronica Aksmanovic, Canadian by birth, with 'Yugoslav' parents, for suggestions on what to see in Slovenia. Her father was raised there, and Veronica put me in touch with her Uncle Tom Lozar in Montreal.

Tom was a fount. If he didn't have an immediate answer to a question he'd have one within a day, with a few added comments. Tom explained that some Slovenians keep bees the way other people keep vineyards, for the simple pleasure of creating an attractive and appealing

376

product. He told me that somewhere he had leftover labels, designed by 'the local Norman Rockwell' under commission from a 'sort of relative' for the 'sort of relative's private honey stash'. In a series of short messages Tom told me that Lojze Peterle, a former Slovenian prime minister and a member of the European parliament was a bee-keeper, that Slovenia's first serious literary magazine in the 1840s was called *Kranjska Čebelica*, or the 'Slovenian Bee', and that, as with the Anglo-Saxons, mead was the favoured drink of ancient Slavs.

Tom suggested that I might want to see how bees are transported to feed on honey and nectar in pastures in Istria and Dalmatia. He told me that in 2003, the World Veterinary Association held a bee-keeping conference in Slovenia and he sent me the programme. After I returned to London and mentioned that my dog enjoyed the *krofi* in Ptuj more than I did, he emailed back, 'The *krofi* you had must have been a bad version. The great ones are of course almost anywhere in Vienna, at Tonolo in Venice (still called *krapfen*, although further south they are called *bombolini*), and, surprise, Café Sbarsky at the Neue Galerie in New York and Café Sicilia in Gloucester, Mass.'

Slovenians have traded in honey and beeswax for at least 600 years and by the 1700s there was a 'Bee-keepers Fraternity', now 'The Bee-keepers Association of Slovenia'. Slovenians are particularly proud of their indigenous, native 'Carniolan' bee and bee-keepers worldwide agree that the Carniolan bee is more docile than others and relatively resistant to disease. It efficiently rears its brood and continues to do so until late in the autumn, as long as food remains available. German bee-keepers have converted completely to Carniolan bees while in the UK, where Italian 'Ligustica' bees augment native 'Mellifera' honeybees in commercial honey-making, especially in southern England, some bee-keepers feel the Slovenian bee should replace both of them.

Carniolan bees are larger than their Italian relatives, with dark, rather than yellow body bands. Breeders say they have a better homing ability than Italian, British or Caucasian bees but that their hybrids—cross-breeds with any other type—are particularly vicious.

In Radovljica, a beautiful little town near Bled, the glazed tile art nouveau decorations on the old bank headquarters showed myriads of bees buzzing industriously. In the fine, rectangular, enclosed and cobbled town square, lined with thickly stuccoed homes on which are variously painted biblical scenes and coats of arms I visited the Museum of Apiculture—the *'Cebelarski Musej'*. What a wonderful place to while away a couple of hours. The museum houses a collection of bee-keepers' materials from historic to present times, and includes a live bee colony, but the highlight—my reason for visiting—was the collection of hundreds of naively painted beehive panels.

Slovenians began painting the fronts of their beehives in the mid-1700s, around the same time they started painting farm furniture. Bee-keepers say the unique images help bees find their own hives more easily. They certainly helped bee-keepers identify individual hives—something that was necessary to remind them which bee colonies had already swarmed and left the hive because all

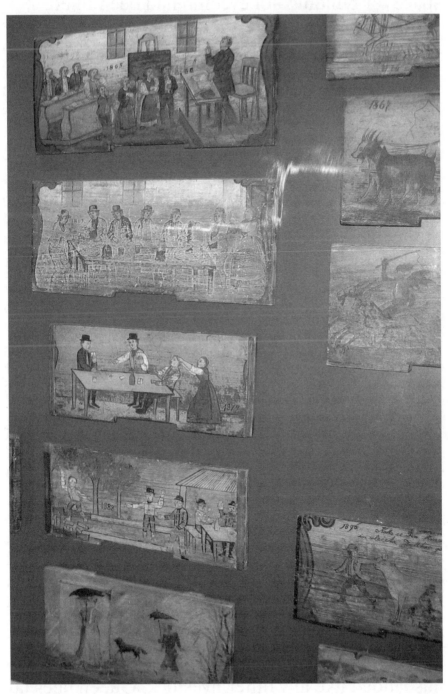

PAINTED BEEHIVE PANELS IN THE APICULTURE
MUSEUM AT RADOVLJICA

space for building honeycomb had been filled.

These paintings are like polychromatic windows into the minds of Slovenian Alpine peasants in the nineteenth century. Early ones portray predominantly religious scenes—copies of church paintings—but by the mid-1800s secular stories and narratives emerged. There are animals, landscapes, and frequently, drawings that ridicule the neighbours, particularly if they're women.

A winged devil, with pliers, holds a woman's tongue to a grindstone. Rabbits carry a dead hunter in a funeral procession, led by a bear reading the Bible, while ducks fly overhead, a deer follows behind carrying the hunter's hat and gun, and the hunter's dog, with head and tail drooped, walks alongside. A snail chases a man. Men carry their wives to a mill although the reason why was lost on me. A bearded man smokes a long pipe while his wife, son and daughter laze around an apiary of nine hives surrounded by buzzing bees. Men drink and play cards around an outdoor table. A husband and wife throw kitchen items at each other. A bear steals a beehive. A bear is shot stealing a beehive. A bear is hunted with dogs.

This is sublime folk art, a true treasure trove. Slovenian bees may have been exported to Britain in these illuminated beehives in Victorian times. I once saw a panel at an antique fair in London, although neither the antique dealer nor I knew at the time the painting came from a Slovenian beehive.

To their owners, bees are livestock, to be husbanded like any other livestock. Queen bees lay eggs, worker bees forage for food and drone bees take care of the hive. Worker bees are born from eggs that are fertilised before the queen lays them—she stores a supply of sperms in her special sac, the spermatheca. If she runs out of sperms she lays unfertilised eggs and these develop into drones.

Old queens eventually become drone-layers, as they say in bee-keeping circles and some clubs in central London. If a colony loses its egg-laying queen bee, worker bees can develop functioning ovaries and start to lay eggs but these are all unfertilised and develop only into drones. Once a colony's workers start laying eggs it's very difficult to 're-queen' it. Bee-keepers either destroy the colony or unite it with another strong one.

Disease risks increase when colonies are united because, just like other livestock, bees are susceptible to infection. Sicknesses affecting immature bees are called 'brood diseases' and the most dangerous are 'foul brood', which is caused by spore-forming bacteria. 'European foul brood' is sometimes treated with antibiotics, although serious infections are treated by burning the colonies and blowtorch-sterilising the hives. The more destructive 'American foul brood' is always treated by killing the bees and sterilising the hive. Antibiotics such as chloramphenicol suppress signs of American foul brood but don't eliminate it and the drugs' residue can end up in honey, so they are usually banned.

'Diseases and the hygiene of bee-keeping' is still a compulsory course for students at The Veterinary Faculty of the University of Ljubljana. They learn bee anatomy, physiology and pathology, how to diagnose and either chemically or biologically treat bee diseases, and they learn about *Varroa destructor*. This aptly named mite originated in Asia and is the bee-keeper's greatest cause of livestock loss. It is prevalent in Slovenia and after it reached the UK in the early 1990s, within 15 years the mite destroyed virtually all wild swarms.

Today, any honey bee you see buzzing in a British garden is almost without doubt from a colony tended by people. There are no wild bees left. When wild or 'feral' colonies re-establish themselves *Varroa destructor* arrives soon after and sucks the life-sustaining bodily fluids from the larvae.

To combat the decline in native bees, British bee-keepers import single queen bees—frequently from Slovenia—usually accompanied by a selection of workers who assiduously provide her with food. On arrival in the UK the workers are killed and the queen is gradually introduced to the members of her new hive. Once she is accepted she sets up a new colony with a selection of hive members. A Slovenian queen bee usually costs around 30 euros but the best can fetch 700 euros.

Today, Slovenian bee-keepers still trundle their beehives to the source of honey and nectar. Honeydew is harvested from chestnut, fir and spruce trees. Nectar is harvested from wild flowers and farm crops. The source of nectar varies from country to country. 'Clover honey' is common in Canada, but Slovene 'blossom honey' today is a mix of honeys from different origins, dandelions, lime trees, clover and buckwheat but also the ubiquitous rape flower.

At the museum shop I bought 450 gram jars of viscous, light brown blossom honey, runny amber-coloured acacia honey, reddish, dark brown, runny spruce honey, green-brown runny silver fir honey and crystallised light brown buckwheat honey, which I later distributed to Veronica and the nurses back at the veterinary clinic.

*   *   *

At 'Camping Bled' at the western end of Lake Bled I returned with a thud to Western tourism. Driving north from Ljubljana towards the majestic snow-touched Julian Alps, I was surrounded, for the first time since my travels began, by squadrons of motorhomes all travelling north in hunting packs. It was off season but there were still over 100 of them at the Bled campgrounds—New Zealanders, British, Dutch, German, French, Italian, Spanish—more than the total number I had seen in all of Scandinavia and Eastern Europe in the last seven weeks.

After checking in, Macy and I walked the pathway around the lake, a two to three-hour walk, past ranks of canopied, seven-metre long, two-metre wide wooden *'pletna'*, the alluring tourist 'gondolas', moored for the night, past strolling Japanese tourists and other dog walkers. The setting was startlingly beautiful, even more so the following morning as I watched the sun appear above the mountains and illuminate the spire of the Church of the Assumption on Bled Island.

The campground was like a kennel: five golden retrievers, four cocker spaniels and various others, all of whom were walked leashed. Cartoon-covered poop bins reminded owners to 'stoop and scoop'. Macy wandered free and other campers

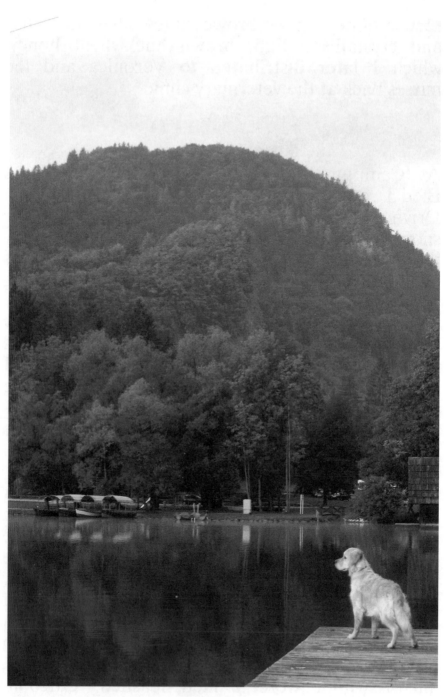

THE CAMPSITE AT LAKE BLED

didn't seem to mind. *'Wunderbar,'* commented a tousle-haired elderly German with a handlebar moustache, *'Ein frei hund.'* I had morning tea with a retired dairy farmer from Rutland.

*   *   *

Julia's plane was arriving in Venice late that afternoon, and impatient to be with her again, I skipped the obvious delights of this beautiful area, rejoined the motorway and through a heavy mist that didn't burn off until late morning headed back south to Ljubljana then west on the A1, towards Trieste. There was one place I wanted to visit before I left, an imposing castle I had last visited in a red Sunbeam Alpine convertible in 1964.

'I drove off the main road on to a ruddy secondary one,' my old diary recounts, 'and from there on to a muddy path, then through someone's barnyard (the chickens had to scramble) along another muddy track until we rounded a bend and suddenly, on the hill before us was the magnificent Predjama Castle, a castle built into a gigantic cave in the side of a cliff.'

Driving up the narrow but now perfectly paved and banked road to Predjama, I stopped in high pasture for a walk and Macy rolled joyously in a field of autumn Alpine crocuses. On my first trip around Europe with my best buddy, a cousin named Calvin, we found a level patch of land nearby and pitched tent for the night. As we got out our sleeping bags we were almost immediately approached by a soldier, a guy our age—around 20. In Spain, when we tried to camp in Catalonia, we'd had guns pointed at us by Civil Guard and

385

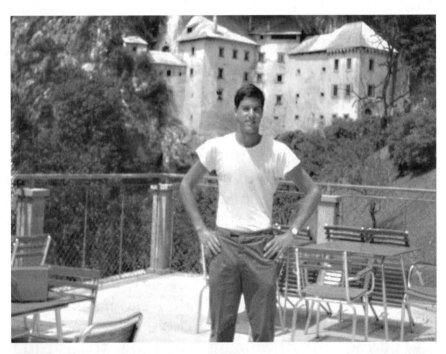

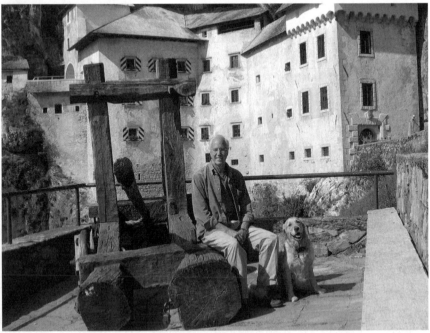

PREDJAMA CASTLE THEN AND NOW

had been told to move on. Here, near Postojna and Predjama, the soldier had offered us his flashlight while we organised ourselves and told us we would be 'safe from gypsies' for the night.

This time, with Macy, there was a coachload of elderly Tyrolean Italians in eagle-feather bedecked, green felt hats visiting when I arrived at Predjama, and in fractured Italian I asked one of them if he would take a photo of Macy and me, with the castle as a backdrop. It would be fun to compare it with a photo Calvin took of me in the same location over 40 years ago.

'*Deutsch?*' he asked and I explained I was '*Inglese—Canadese.*'

'*Inglese!*' he repeated to me and then to his comrades and I got a double handshake and a gap-toothed smile and incomprehensible jokes about Macy. Before I could ask who they were the men quickstepped back to their tour bus and departed.

*   *   *

On the A3 motorway, a few miles from the Italian border, I passed a road sign to Lipica. It was Uncle Tom Lozar who had suggested I visit Lipica where a 'Society of Friends of Lipica', founded by a Slovenian poet, Boris A Novak, was trying to prevent 50 hectares of the Lipizzaner horses' pastureland, one sixth of its land, being turned into an 18-hole golf course.

'Slovenians claim the Lipizzaner horses as their own, since Lipica (the original spelling) was a village in (Austro-Hungarian) Slovenia.' Tom explained in another parenthesis-riddled email. To emphasise his point he quoted a stanza from an

387

Edvard Kocbek poem called *Lipicanci*, translated by him into English.

> Others have reverenced sacred cows and
>   dragons,
> millennial turtles and lions with wings,
> two-headed eagles, unicorns, and the phoenix;
> we chose the loveliest beast of all:
> it proved its mettle in circuses and battle,
> transported princesses and monstrances all
>   gold,
> and that is why, though the Emperor in Vienna
> spoke French to canny diplomats;
> Italian, to the latest ingenue;
> Spanish, to the eternal God;
> and German, with the untutored help;
> to his horses, he always spoke Slovenian.

Tom promised he'd get in touch with Professor Novak who had written a play soon to be performed for the first time at the Municipal Theatre in Ljubljana, *Lipizzans go to Strasbourg* in which two stallions and a mare called Europa go to the European Court of Human Rights in Strasbourg where they file a complaint against the human race. The court decides to hear the case and the horses call witnesses—Maria Theresa, Napoleon, General Patton, Marshal Tito—to explain the history of horses.

I couldn't stop to see the stud now—Julia's plane was arriving at Marco Polo Airport in only a few hours and with a little regret I drove on past it and a few kilometres on, reached the border and crossed back into 'Old Europe', to a language I recognised, a food I loved, and a culture I felt

388

comfortable in. It was like a homecoming.

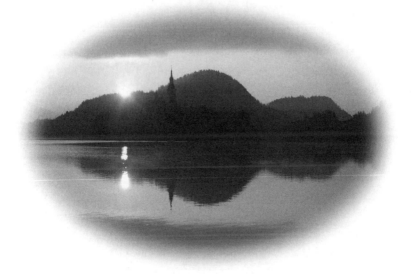

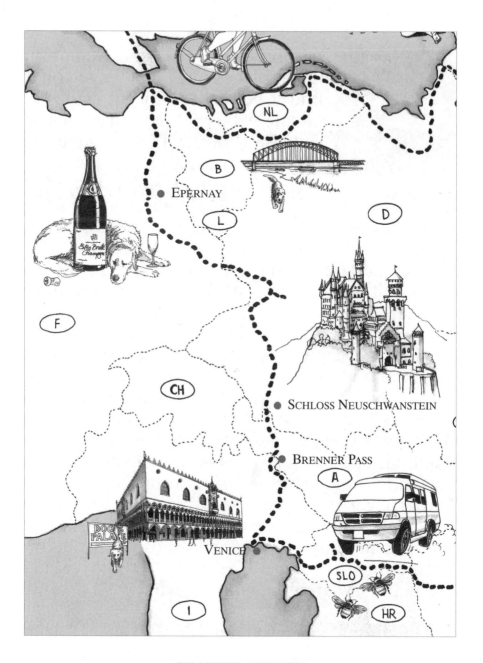

CHAPTER ELEVEN

THROUGH OLD EUROPE

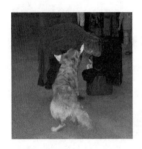 Airports are frenetic, emotion-laden places but I challenge you to find a better way to put smiles on people's faces than, in a sea of suitcases, have a large blonde dog suddenly recognise her favourite, best in the whole wide world, small blonde woman. Normally undemonstrative, Macy squealed with joyous glee and danced with delight when she recognised Julia amongst the torrent of tourists at Marco Polo Airport. Her wagging tail air-conditioned the whole hall. My dog and my wife left the terminal arm in arm and, outside, I got a chance to squeeze Julia too.

The landscape on the drive to the airport had been flat and orderly—rows of cypress and poplar trees stretched south towards the sea; to the north, were regimented vineyards, with climbing pink roses decorating the front of each row of grape-laden vines. Although it was mid-October, it was hot and muggy. On the drive from the Slovenian border, over the top of the Adriatic to Venice, big gooey bugs had left their sticky impressions on the windscreen and I cleaned those off before continuing to Venice. Macy and I both calmed down and updated the chief on what we'd recently seen and done.

The three of us walked from Tronchetto, an artificial island built to hold a multi-storey car park, to the Rialto Bridge. Bad move. The heat washed away Julia's energy, and the sea of legs that Macy had to negotiate intimidated her. The crowded *vaporetto* ride down the Grand Canal was

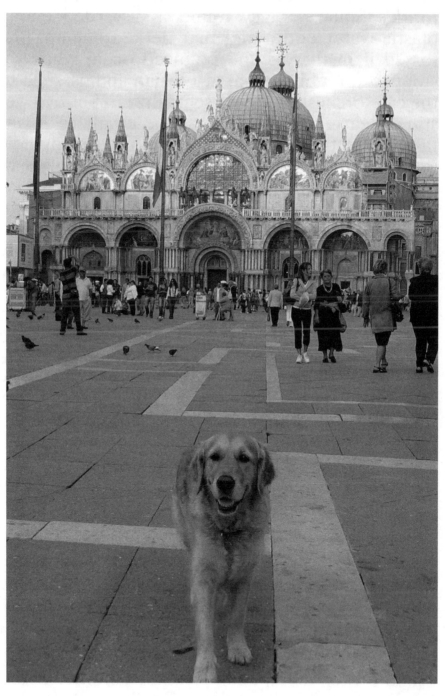

THE BASILICA OF ST. MARK THE EVANGELIST,
VENICE

no better. We were like sardines in oil. In St. Mark's Square, Macy found a discarded empty plastic water bottle and that perked her up. She tossed it in the air and pounced on it, while we stopped for a bite to eat at Florian and listened to the café orchestra play its schmaltzy, repetitive, yet still endearingly delightful Viennese waltzes. It was fascinating to see how Macy could fit her by now extremely large tongue into a very small glass of Florian water, in order to have a drink.

Julia and I know Venice well. We visit yearly and stay with friends, who were away this weekend. We'd planned to have dinner at Alla Madonna by the Rialto, where we'd once been entertained by the visiting Swedish all-male choir, then to drive back to one of the campsites we'd passed between the airport and the causeway, but the heat and the crowds were oppressive and we decided to skip the meal. Back at Tronchetto, our patch of tarmac by the edge of the lagoon, under a line of bird-filled trees, seemed far better situated than any campsite we would find. Besides, we'd been apart for a long time and wanted to get to know each other once more, sooner rather than later, so we camped in Venice for the night.

*　　　*　　　*

By 7 a.m. the first coffee kiosk had received its delivery of croissants, had brewed up and opened. I sat under the trees overlooking the lagoon and had breakfast. Mosquitoes had returned overnight, squadrons of them, and Julia was tentative about leaving the security of the Roadtrek. I cooked breakfast for her and, as the bloodsuckers hovered outside the camper's screens, humming invective at her, we decided to depart for the mainland, and higher ground.

Do you know that even Euro-songs sound better in Italian? I can't tell you how much I enjoyed being back in a land I felt familiar with. Part of that delight came from vaguely understanding a little of the language; it also derives from a familiarity with the culture, a form of intimacy that evolves through previous encounters.

At Conegliano we drove up the narrow road to the castellated, manicured, hilltop castle, which we had to ourselves. Macy saw it as her responsibility to control the feral cat population while I saw it as my responsibility to see whether I could pocket a ripe pomegranate from one of the trees. Julia reined us both in. Party over. The chief was back and we were both put on short leads.

We drove on north, along old roads lined with walnut trees, past the faded blue waters of Lago di Sante Croce, into the Pieve river valley, to Pieve di Cadore and the Dolomites.

The lands we were driving through are not covered in my 1913 *Baedeker's Northern Italy* because this region was part of Austria until the massive land redistributions that occurred after World War One, when the province was assigned to Italy. We were back, once more, under the influence of Mitteleuropa. In Cortina d'Ampezzo, which nests in a sun-catching, cross-shaped meadow surrounded by a ring of majestic mountains we stopped for a quick and uninspiring lunch. I bought *fraises de bois* for Julia to nibble on and a jar of almost black, spruce honey for my honey collection, from a grocer who looked like an elegant, elderly, aristocrat selling produce from his estate.

The Alto Adige-Sud Tirol region we continued through is mostly German-speaking, although interestingly, my 1899 *Baedeker's Austria-Hungary* says 'The language spoken is "Ladin" but German is generally understood.' Today, only four per cent of local people speak Ladin, a strange blend of Latin and mountain Celtic, a remnant language left behind by the Roman soldiers sent here to pacify the local Celts 1500 years ago.

We continued through the lazy Rienza river valley, dotted with bilingually named, Tyrolean towns—Monguelfo/Welsberg, Brunico/Bruneck and Vandoies/Vinti, then on to the motorway from Bolzano/Bolzen up to the 1375 metre-high Brenner Pass, the lowest pass over the Alps, into Austria itself.

We didn't linger long there; my run of good weather had broken, and now it was raining steadily, and the mosquitoes were vigorously alert. We crossed the narrow 'panhandle' of the Austrian Tyrol which reaches west to Switzerland and drove rapidly on north-west into Germany and across Bavaria.

We had a quick pit-stop at the fairytale Schloss Neuschwanstein, King Ludwig II's phantasmic recreation of a medieval German castle, and the inspiration for Walt Disney's fantasyland confection. Dogs weren't allowed inside, so I walked Macy in the nearby woods, and from above the trees, like a mirage in a desert, the turrets of the castle emerged, and soon, the entire, enticing structure. Cotton white, misty clouds formed and reformed around it. It was like the most dramatic

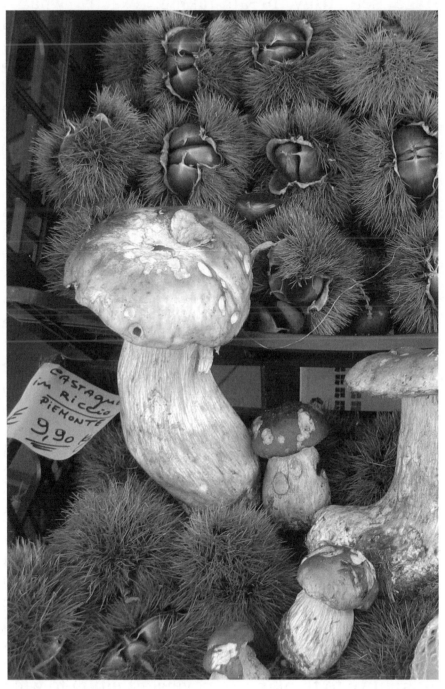

MUSHROOMS AND CHESTNUTS FOR SALE IN CORTINA D'AMPEZZO

stage set, truly breath-taking, exactly what I imagine the weird and wonderful Ludwig II wanted it to be.

As we left Bavaria for Baden-Württemberg we stuck to the *autobahns*, whizzing past castles and museums and 'points of interest', camping overnight at Heidelberg where, the next day, we visited a veterinary clinic. Macy had to be treated once more for ticks, as UK law stipulates, by any vet in the entire universe other than me, who would sign her documents for her return to the UK. At Mannheim we crossed the Rhine and drove on to Kaiserslauten, then Saarbrucken and into France: the home straight.

Rain was still falling as we drove west through France, past Metz and Châlons-en-Champagne to the hills of Reims and to Epernay, on the south bank of the Marne. We booked ourselves into the Royal Champagne Hotel, to an expansive room with its own terrace overlooking the vineyard-covered hills of the valley to the south. Luxury after weeks in the Roadtrek. Julia, Macy and I were invited to sit down by the fire in the long drawing-room and have champagne and some truly scrumptious madeleine biscuits, before being shown our room.

It had been a good trip, an excellent one, not necessarily the journey I had expected but one in which favourable weather had allowed me to get a feel for the countryside of the 'neglected' eastern regions of Europe. Of course I took countless photos and hope I didn't used my camera as an alternative to thinking, to paying attention to what I saw.

For me, travel fills a personal need to step

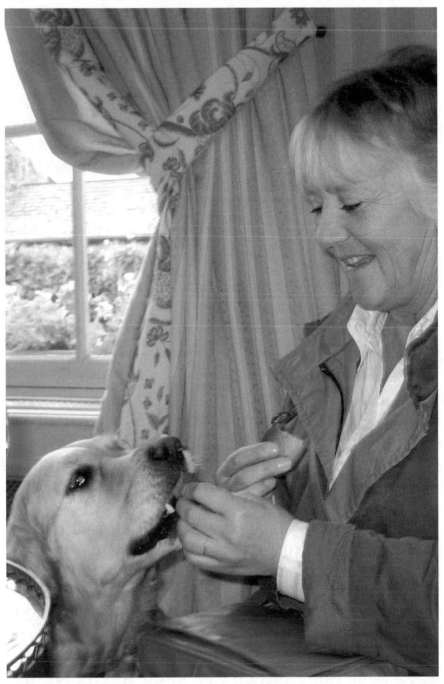

Madeleine biscuits at the Royal Champagne
Hotel

outside of my own daily routines, not just to say that I've 'been there, done that', but to refresh my senses, to capture more textures of life. The experiences of greatest value are the most beautiful ones and while some of these are made by us, many are part of nature, or of nature's interaction with what we have made. What I find rewarding is not just aesthetic beauty but also the beauty of function, of performance, of consequence: how a bee colony works; how mushrooms grow; how Lars Vilks' columns at Nimis survive winter storms; how water makes patterns when it laps on smooth rock; how a stork makes a nest; how light changes at dusk; how people adapt to their surroundings; how the cycle of life continues.

Writing about what I see is my way of noticing rather than just looking, of securing my memories. The Great European Plain, where I spent most of my time, is visually uninspiring. There's no drama to it. It's easy to miss its beauty. Worse, it's been blighted by its recent, and foul, Soviet occupation. But when the region is noticed rather than looked at, it is unarguably beautiful in its own subtle, even enigmatic way.

This journey also exposed me to realities I'd prefer not to think about. At home, at work, there are always incessant demands. Life is so full, it's easy to avoid challenging internal conversations, to restrict yourself to simple, practical, easy thoughts. But when you travel alone, your internal emotional censor, that part of you that clamps a lid on things when something difficult is about to emerge into your mind, into your consciousness, goes on holiday.

*　　　*　　　*

When I set out on this trip I intended to visit 'new Europe', to see what people were doing and planning, but the only way to begin to understand Eastern Europe is to acknowledge that it's a product of its past. That was an uncomfortable experience for me. By travelling through the eastern regions of Europe I was forced to confront the lurking, dark core of human behaviour, ever waiting to be unleashed from the confines of social order. I worry that, while countries such as Germany have been exemplary in confronting their painful history in an honest and forthright manner, there are swathes of 'new Europe' that are still in denial. People say, 'He was like an animal,' when a man has acted cruelly and callously, but there is no animal more capable of cruelty and depravity than us.

*　　　*　　　*

Julia and I celebrated and had Bellinis and a bottle of pink champagne with our meal. While I chatted on about aspects of the trip, Julia picked up her bread plate and, as all antique dealers do, checked out where it was made and who made it.

'Oh look. It's Limoges!' she smiled, her eyes twinkling at her discovery that the dinner-service porcelain was from her favourite 'china town'.

It was no more than a natural comment, a happily discovered fact, a recognition that we were eating in a classy restaurant, but the sound of the word 'Limoges' was like a rifle shot. I felt cold. I

401

lost my hunger. 'Limoges.' Such a beautiful word. If I hadn't gone on this trip it still would be just that; a word that brings to mind beauty, refinement, sophistication, elegance, glory, culture—gentility. Limoges has a new meaning I can't erase. Such a banal statement: 'We are 500 Frenchmen from Limoges.'

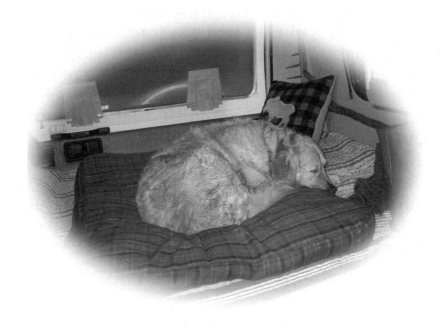

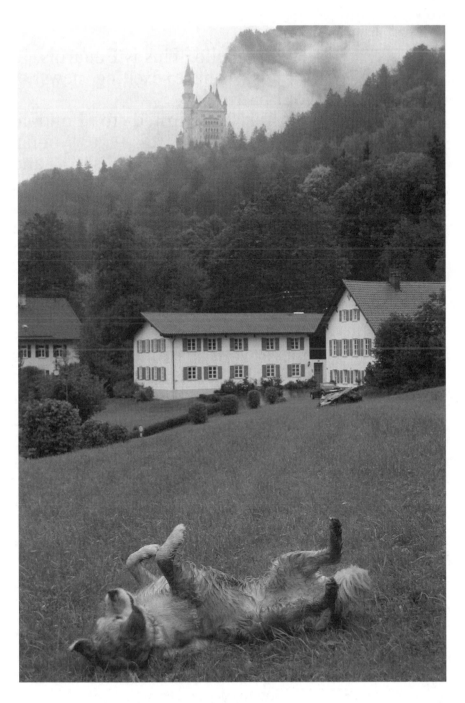

EPILOGUE

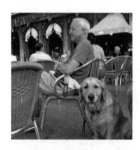

'Hello? Hello. This is Eduardis. In Vilnius. I have exciting news of your patrimony.'

After I returned to London, I hired Eduardis, a young, entrepreneurial, Polish and Russian-reading, Lithuanian genealogist to scour old archive records housed in Vilnius, to see if he could discover exactly where in that benighted land the Fogles and Bernards once lived.

'My researches are very positive. I believe I find cheerful evidence that your family has connections with Hollywood!' he continued. 'Early in my researches I believe your patrimonial name is Fikhel,' he went on, 'I discovered several Fikhels lived in the Kaunas region in the 1860s, but Dr Fogle I do not believe they are your ancestors. After further extensive researches using all the names you give me I believe that you are truly a Fuckoff.'

I know I have the ability to irritate people, but I thought that the sheer number of euros I was slipping into Eduardis' bank account would lubricate our relationship. This wasn't exactly what I wanted to hear. Eduardis continued, with rising excitement in his voice.

'What is more wonderful is that my researches discover that the great Hollywood actor, Mr Columbo, his father also came from the same administrative district as your grandfather. He too was a Fuckoff but when he moved to America he became a simple Fuck. Peter Fuck is one of your relatives!'

I can't tell you how relieved I was to hear this. To help Eduardis, I'd given him the surnames of all my Scottish relatives from the 1880s, Glasgow family tree: Fogle and Bernard, but also Lann, Ross, Sender, Riffkin, Rosenberg, Hirsch, Dykes, Elkin, Naftalin and Abbott, which I knew had been anglicised from Abramovich. Amongst the list of names was one of my great-great-grandmothers, Minnie Falcoff.

'Eduardis, how do you spell my family surname?' I asked.

'F-A-L-C-K-O-F-F. I do not find evidences for any of the people in the genealogy list you give me, but I am sure you are a Fuckoff because I find no records for Fogle in any spelling in the national archives for Kovno Guberniya. I believe your family are Fuckoffs in Lithuania and change their name to Fogle, just as the father of Peter Fuck was once a Fuckoff and he changed his name when he moved to America. You know Bruce, what is most exciting is I thought Peter Fuck was Italian. Mr Columbo is Lithuanian, from Kaunas!'

Eduardis' research into the Fogle name had hit a brick wall. The Falcoffs were a completely different branch of the family, becoming the Phillips in Canada, where a distant relative of mine, Nathan Phillips, was mayor of Toronto when I was a boy. There may still be records somewhere in the archives of the Russian Imperial Province of Kovno Guberniya, of the Fogle and Bernard families, living in the same town or village, but too many generations have now passed for any in the family to know the name of the district or village— the *uyezd* or *shtetl*—vital information for tracing exactly where they lived and what they did.

*   *   *

My DNA analysis was more fruitful. After I returned home I had a cheek swab analysed at the same lab in New Mexico—DNA Tribes—where my cousin Erik had his analysed. DNA Tribes offers a generalised 'World Region Match' with scores over 1.0 indicating a genetic affinity to world regions. I scored:

Mediterranean	5.77
North-west European	4.11
Mestizo (people of mixed Hispanic/North American native ancestry)	3.26
Eastern European	3.26
North African	2.27
Arabian	2.18
Asia Minor	2.04

With the exception of his primary Finno-Ugrian world region match, Erik, with whom I have 25 per cent of my DNA in common, had a similar score. If that's correct, it suggests that some of our ancestors might have migrated out of 'Asia Minor'—the region from the Caucasus through Mesopotamia to the Mediterranean—and Arabia, through Northern Africa to the European side of the Mediterranean where they lived for a protracted time, then on to North-west Europe where they also lived for an extended period, and finally to where I know they lived, in Eastern Europe, where their residence was probably shorter.

The genetics lab provided me with my own 'Native Population Match', comparing my DNA with over 400 native populations that have experienced little change in the last 500 years. These results gave me clues to my deep ancestral origins. My top 10 DNA matches were:

Bavarian (Germany)	57.7
Portuguese	24.2
Minorcan (Spain)	19.1
Russian	15.7
Macedonian	15.4
Basque	15.2
Balearic Islands (Spain)	14.7
Northern Portuguese	14.7
Andalusian (Spain)	13.3
Flemish	13.0

So all those people who asked *'Deutsch?'* when I met them were partly right! It looks like I share more DNA with the native population of southern Germany than with any other geographical group, and large portions with people from throughout Spain and Portugal. The impressive Moorish synagogue I saw in Lesko, built in 1643 as part of the town's defences, is superb evidence that Spanish and Portuguese Jews had certainly settled in the south-west corner of Poland by the early 1600s. I knew my Dutch Uncle Bram could trace his origins back to Portugal and Spain, because of his surname, 'Eriera', and now I have genetic evidence that some of my ancestors probably made a similar journey from the Iberian peninsula to the Baltic, perhaps via southern Germany.

Finally, DNA Tribes provided me with a comparison to 567 global populations, as they are today as a result of recent migrations and admixtures rather than the 'native population' who had been in place for longer periods. My DNA is still most similar to Bavaria's present-day population than to any other and these results also confirm that the Iberian Peninsula—Portugal and Spain—is the region of the Mediterranean where my ancestors bred. The top 10 results are:

Bavarian (Germany)	57.7
Caucasian	29.5
Portuguese	24.2
Bocaya, Colombia	23.0
Maracaibo, Venezuela	21.2
Hispanic New York	20.9
Hispanic	20.4
Minorcan (Spain)	19.1
Caucasian (Indiana)	18.8
Caucasian (Canada)	18.1

This was so much fun I arranged for my 92-year-old mother, the last of her generation, to have her DNA analysed. Her highest 'Native Population Matches' were Spanish and Bavarian-German, but sandwiched between the two was Norway. My mother is a natural blonde, with hazel eyes. Is this genetic evidence that there was an unauthorised alliance between one of her ancestors and a visiting Viking? Her added Nordic bloodline gives her a slightly different 'World Region Match' to mine. Hers is:

North-west European	8.41
Mediterranean	8.07
Mestizo	5.85
Asia Minor	4.59
Eastern European	4.45

I gave my results to one of my Scottish Bernard relatives who had his DNA analysed and discovered his World Region Match was mostly North-west European, Eastern European and Finno-Ugrian, with much less Mediterranean matching. Neither he nor my mother had Portuguese (or North African or Arabian) matches so those of mine probably come from my father's father's side. The accuracy of all these results, of course, depends wholly on the mathematical algorithm the analysts use. Who knows how accurate they really are, but it's so much fun comparing them. My wife and children are next.

*   *   *

Soon after we returned from our travels I became much more interested in Macy's DNA. Macy's right eye started to go wrong. It got 'slow', then her third eyelid, the nictitating membrane, became more prominent. It relaxed until it covered her eyeball, preventing her from seeing on her right side. Her right upper lid drooped so much she looked like she had a horrible headache. This is a condition called Horner's Syndrome, rare, but a known genetic glitch in some golden retrievers. Fortunately, although the cause isn't known, it usually affects only one eye and in most instances spontaneously resolves itself within six months.

Macy was different. Within weeks, her left eye started to show the first signs of similar changes. This wasn't going to be a simple Horner's for she was also developing a bilateral 'strabismus', with the muscles in her right eye pulling that one down and to the right and those in her left eye pulling that one up and to the right. Only the whites of her eyes were visible and both eyeballs were slowly sinking back into their sockets. Then she developed a head tilt.

Something was affecting five different cranial nerves and the common denominator for those various nerves was her brain, so I arranged for a veterinary neurologist to thoroughly examine her and carry out an MRI brain scan. The scan revealed she did have a brain and, more importantly, eliminated the possibility of a brain tumour.

I had her checked for any nasty, Continental, tick-borne diseases too, feeling a surge of guilt, but she was clear. Other than becoming blind and cocking her head quizzically, she was healthy, and coping far better with her disabilities than either Julia or I were. Her condition was 'idiopathic', a word Julia has come to hate.

Surgically removing both third eyelids temporarily restored some vision to her right eye. Being a dog and not dwelling on what once was, she adapted well, walking with her head turned up towards the heavens and to the left so she could see ahead out of the bottom right corner of her right eye, but her eyeballs continued to sink into their sockets and now the lids rolled inside out and her lashes started to ulcerate her eyes. More surgery, removing lots of skin above and below her eyes, stopped further damage and once more gave her limited vision. Julia was pleased with Macy's eye job and asked whether vets offered the same service to dog owners.

Macy will need more surgery in the future and her successful hunting days are now over. Squirrels stick their tongues out at her and continue foraging on the ground, but she's modified her hunting tactics and listens for rustling rather than watching for movement. She's not bad, but now she charges off to the left when she hears rustling, arcing back to the right, towards the source of the sound, too late for success. It's heartbreaking.

Macy's travelling days are over. Journeying was always boring to her and now, with limited sight, letting her run off in strange places—always risky—is impossible. If I ever go travelling extensively through Europe again and want a canine companion, I do have a few other family possibilities, all of whom love motor travel. There's my daughter's hyperkinetic, black Labrador, Lola, my son Ben's goofy black Lab Inca (Lola's mother), and his wife Marina's razor-sharp, chocolate-coloured Lab-Border collie-cross, Maggi.

Ben and Marina wanted me to drive Inca and Maggi, through whom they met while walking their dogs in the park, to Monsaraz in Portugal when they married there. I liked the idea. The interior of Portugal remains even now isolated by its remoteness from the rest of Europe and there are unique regional dog breeds, such as the Estrella Mountain Dog, bred in out-of-the-way villages.

There are ghost towns in these mountains, ancient villages abandoned in the 1970s for economic reasons. Surprisingly, in the mountain town of Belmonte, lives one of Portugal's largest Jewish communities—over 120 families.

After the Inquisition of 1492, most families fled, many to Holland, others to Germany or further, to south-eastern Poland. Those who stayed agreed to convert to Christianity. For the next 480 years, outwardly Catholic, they practised their Jewish faith in secret.

It was only after the 1974 Portuguese Revolution that they felt secure enough to profess their beliefs. Ten years ago, the first synagogue to be built in Portugal for almost 500 years was opened on the site of the house where they had secretly prayed for over 20 generations. That story has a bit more piquancy, now that I know I share some of my DNA with the Portuguese. I wonder whether magical Maggi, my bright, new, dog-in-law, would like to step into Macy's paw tracks?

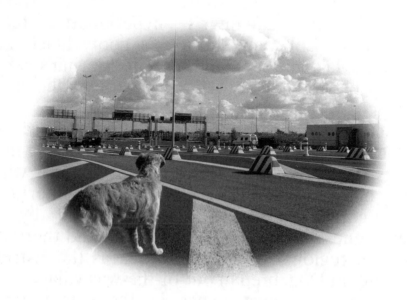

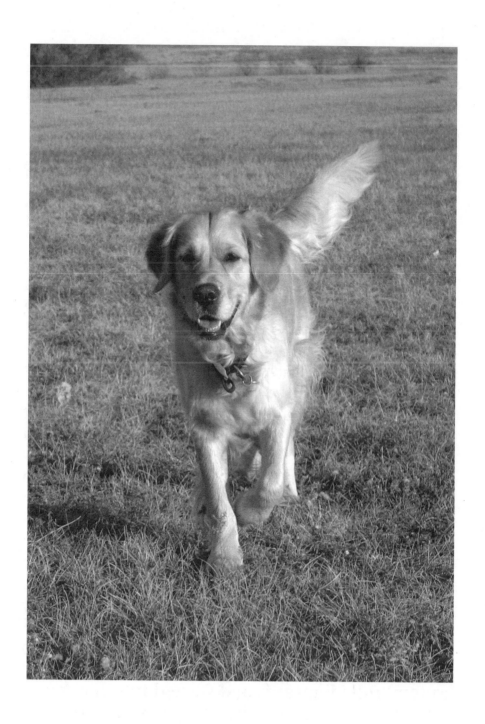

POSTSCRIPT

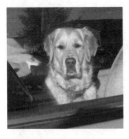My dog Macy certainly travelled extensively and people who read of our activities routinely asked where we were going next. I'd have to explain we weren't going anywhere, not because I didn't want to travel any more with her but because, although she was only six years old, she'd lost most of her sight.

At first one of her eyes simply started to wander, to drop down and to the right. She had a condition called Horner's Syndrome, something that when it happens to a golden retriever almost always affects only one eye. The condition usually spontaneously resolves within six months. But Macy's eye looked different. It had 'wandered' more than a typical Horner's. And it didn't spontaneously resolve. Instead, within weeks a similar problem started to develop in her other eye. The muscles in that eye pulled the eyeball up and to the right. And her head tilted quizzically to the left, another condition called 'vestibular syndrome'.

With five separate cranial nerves no longer functioning properly and her third eyelids permanently drooped over her eyeballs, surgically removing those membranes temporarily restored some vision. But both eyes continued to sink into their sockets and soon all of her eyelids, top and bottom, rolled inwards and started to ulcerate her eyeballs. I've been in veterinary practice for over 35 years and had never seen anything like it. A brain scan and cerebrospinal fluid tap both proved negative for specific causes of her condition. I arranged for an ophthalmic veterinary surgeon friend to remove lots of skin around her eyes and that saved her eyeballs, restoring vision to one of them, her right eye. If the sun wasn't shining too brightly, her right pupil dilated enough for her to see well enough to avoid crashing into trees.

One of the unalloyed joys of the trips I'd taken with Macy was the satisfaction I got from seeing her—letting her—be a free-thinking dog. Yes, I know that's not how we're supposed to behave with our dogs. We're supposed to 'control' them. But Macy's free-thinking travels were now over and I was reconciled to exercising her only in places where it was safe to do so. And then, suddenly and unexpectedly, she died. I'd accommodated to her being effectively blind but this was an earth-shaker. If you're a dog owner you'll understand how I felt.

During my married life I've had three previous dogs, all of whom got well into their double digits. I shed a few tears when each of them died, but somehow Macy's death was a more painful stab in the heart. For catharsis I wrote down how I felt and a few months later went back to what I'd written and submitted it to *The Independent*. They published it, as did the *Daily Mail* the following day, to a greater and more emotional response than any newspaper article I'd previously written.

This is what I wrote.

DOG GONE: MOURNING A PET

Why do sensible, level-headed people find the death of a pet so hard to cope with? Recently

415

bereaved vet Bruce Fogle reflects on the complicated, and often heartbreaking, relationship between a man and his best friend.

I'm unanchored. Emotionally adrift. Not because my marriage has hit the skids, or because my children are unwell. I haven't lost my job. I'm not even moving home. My mind's in a stew for a banal, some of you might say a really trivial, reason: my dog died.

It's not that my dog was anything particularly special. She was a family dog, a six-year-old female golden retriever, one of the umpteen dogs you might see every day being exercised by their owners. But she was my dog, a warm, soft, beautiful, loving thing.

Macy was a thoughtful creature, a considerate being, a trusting and worthy part of my family. She was also my travelling companion, accompanying me on long travels we took together around North America and New Europe.

There are some, and you may be one, who dislike the anthropomorphising of dogs: the humanising of their personalities, their feelings, their emotions. To me, there are shades of this. I hate seeing dogs in party hats or wearing antlers at Christmas. But can you seriously refuse to grant a dog the complexities of emotional feelings? Many do, but I can't accept that. I can't believe that dogs don't have emotions and the only words I have to describe those emotions are ones I'd use to describe a fellow human.

My dog Macy was 'jealous' when another dog took one of her toys, 'thoughtful' before trying anything unfamiliar, 'joyous' when she met people or other dogs she knew, 'contented' to be left alone, 'purposeful' when investigating the natural world around her, 'circumspect' in her approach to

416

unknown people, 'contained' in her display of emotions. Helen Mirren in The Queen reminded me of Macy—guarded, wary, restrained, but no less 'human' for it.

But there's a trickier emotion. Can you describe love? Can you put your own feeling of love for someone into precise words? Can you capture in a sentence or a paragraph that feeling of love so that someone reads and understands what you mean?

I know the look of love in my wife's eyes, but can I describe in words what that look is? (I know, too, her look of exasperation, or annoyance.) You can't dispassionately describe love from the outside. You have to feel it from the inside in order to know what it is, so you'll have to take my word for it. As trite as it may sound, I loved my dog and I know my dog loved me.

Why do we love a species that so depends on us? We guide our kids from their early reliance on us to eventual independence, but the dog's dependence is permanent and we love them deeply for it. An evolutionary biologist would say that's the dog's trump card—her ability to convince us that she needs us for ever and ever. They thrive on our lifelong need to nurture.

Macy did this in a number of ways. First, there was that look in her eyes. It was exactly the same as the look of love in my wife's eyes. So why is it any different from the love Julia need not put into words?

There's another look she could get in her eyes— absolute, unmitigated, concentrated interest in me. An uncle of mine had that look and women generations younger than he fell in love with him because of it. So why can't I fall in love with that look in my dog's eyes, a look that told me she

417

thought I was the most interesting and vital person she'd ever met?

Then there's physical contact. Golden retrievers are particularly adept at this. They press their bodies into you. Each time I returned home, Macy pressed her head against my legs when she greeted me. Sometimes she did this in the park, too. Just because. If I were sitting, on a chair or in the grass, she'd come over and press her chest against me. It's as if she were saying: 'I want to squeeze you I love you so much, and this is the best I can do.'

And silence. Is that not the true glue of love: the ability to be together, to do together, to understand each other without the need for words? The ability to feel love certainly pre-dates language. Being with a dog, understanding her moods, her wants, her feelings, her emotions, without the need for words, returns you to the core of your being, to a time before words, when body language said everything.

As so many dogs do, Macy bestowed unconditional devotion, an unquestioning reliability, a constancy and an immutability. Her intention was always to be there, to leaven anywhere with the familiarity of her presence. After the thrill of the chase, even when lost in the deepest woods, her purpose was always to return, to find me, to be rejoined once more. Of course, that's at the core of the most sentimental stories about dogs. Every culture has them: the dog awaiting his master's return, even from the dead. That's unmitigated sentiment but, I ask you, what's wrong with that? Can another human ever equal the unqualified, unconditional regard that a dog has for us?

Living with a dog is an ongoing process of interpreting. We intuitively interpret what our dogs, with their bodies, tell us, and when we can't fully interpret we take them to the vet so that he interprets what's happening. As well as her owner, I was also Macy's vet. I'm used to that triangular relationship, you, your dog and me, all interacting with each other.

I usher dogs through life, from the faltering first steps of puppyhood, through the arc of life to the often pain-riddled last steps of stoic old age. I have a relationship with the dog and with her owner. To dogs, I provide medical care. To owners, I offer experience and advice. There are times when I have to cut myself loose from the emotional link I've made with my patient and speak dispassionately with her owner. 'Are we doing such and such because it's good for the dog or are we doing it because we can't bear the emotional torment of the only alternative: to painlessly kill.' But when it's my own dog that's gravely ill, there's no triad. Who do I talk to about her?

Walking your dog is life-affirming and it's probably what I miss most now that she's no longer alive. It's as if you're plaited together, one extended consciousness, awareness overlapping. I see a squirrel before she does, and then she spies one before I do. On one of those walks, rather than charging ahead in front of me, Macy unexpectedly walked beside me. Dogs develop ritual behaviours and, because Macy had deviated from hers, there in the park I examined her and felt a mass the size of a chicken egg, fixed firm in her guts.

I pretended to myself, and later to my wife Julia, that it was an ovarian cyst but knew that was unlikely. I took her to the clinic, withdrew a blood sample and found nothing unexpected but I knew I'd have to operate to see what the mass was.

That night, in obvious distress, Macy came to Julia's side of our bed and, with anxiety in her eyes, she panted relentlessly. I gave her a painkiller and she relaxed but it wasn't until the following morning, when I operated on her, that I knew for certain that she had haemorrhaged in her abdomen. Once the blood was cleared away I found the site of her bleeding and removed it. There were other sites too, filled with cheesy material, like pus but not pus, and I removed most of them too. But not all of them. There were simply too many.

Veronica and I operated for three hours, removing large parts of her innards. Veronica worked in emergency and critical care in California before she joined me in London, but neither of us was absolutely certain what we were dealing with. After we finished surgery and Veronica took off her face mask, I saw in her eyes what her mind was thinking: 'Poor Macy. Poor Bruce.' What was in my mind was: 'Why have I operated?'

Four days later, we got back the results from the pathologist. A wickedly fast-spreading cancer that had originated somewhere on her skin had invaded all her organs, spreading in sheets around healthy tissue. The cheesy material was nothing more than tissue that had lost its blood supply and died.

When we finished operating, I still didn't know the exact cause of her condition but experience told me that whatever it was, her life would be short and probably uncomfortable. I didn't want to lose my dog but I didn't want her to wake up either. I increased the narcotic painkiller and took her home to Julia. There, I continued to add painkiller to her intravenous drip and, lying by the sofa, conscious but asleep, by the light of the fire, she died that evening, not having had the distress of re-awakening.

Just that week I'd received a book from an American publisher, hoping that I'd write a blurb for the back jacket. It was an intelligent and attractive tale, told by Ted Kerasote, a self-sufficient outdoorsman from Wyoming, of his life with a big yellow dog named Merle. Of course, every book about a dog tells the story of its end.

Of Merle's end of life, Ted wrote: 'Rocking back on my heels I wondered how this could be—his going off while I was cleaning his butt. Somehow, it seemed apt. A dog is always more interested in another dog's rear end than in its eyes. Half laughing, half crying at this thought, I suddenly felt all my joints lose cohesion, as if what had been holding me together had suddenly dissolved. "My dog," I said to the empty house. "My dog."'

Ted only had his empty house. I had Julia and, although we didn't need words, we too dissolved. When dogs are members of the family, when we know they have feelings and emotions so similar to ours, when we grieve for their passing as we do for any other beings we have formed bonds with, we need rituals to help us cope with the end of a life. Julia and I stayed with her body for a while, my fingers buried in my dog's hair for my comfort now rather than for hers, then I wrapped her in a sheet, put her on her bed in the back of the car and drove to Sussex.

At dawn the next morning, I started digging under a low, bushy bay tree where on hot days she had silently retreated for shade. The clay was as hard as concrete but this was a satisfying ritual I'd carried out before. I've got two more dogs, Liberty and Lex, buried in their favourite spots in that garden. It's a final service, a last 'thank you' to an innocent. Rigor mortis had come and gone and as I carried her from the car to the hole I'd dug, her head lolled like a flower on an old stem. Mock me if you must, but I buried with her all the lost tennis balls that she'd found in the park during the previous month and proudly carried back to the car, 11 of them.

Dogs can't tell their life stories, but sentimentally, and I dare say tediously, we dog owners tend to narrate our dogs' lives to others. To those who have not formed an emotional bond with an individual dog, a description of the quiet intimacies in that relationship can be discomfiting. To those of you who have, let me say this, both from my own experience and from watching so many others endure the grief of losing a dog.

What differentiates the loss of a dog from the loss of a fellow human is the fact that the core values in our affiliation with dogs can be re-formed. The emotional value of living in the company of a dog does not reside solely and uniquely within that one individual. A dog dies and that particular dog is irreplaceable, but the value of 'dog' can be filled by others.

Macy was the fourth dog we've had during our marriage, and certainly the most travelled. I've surprised myself by how cut up I still feel about her premature death. Maybe that's because she died young, or because I spent so many months on the road, travelling alone with her, sharing experiences with her and no one else. Or maybe it's because she was my first 'digital dog'. It seems that every time my screensaver comes on there's another random picture of Macy, among lingonberries on the Russian border, ploughing through the surf of an empty Oregon beach, at Florian's café in Venice. The memories *remain, but I know too that, inevitably and joyously, she will soon be followed by a fifth.*

*   *   *

And so she was. Six months later LL Bean, an eight-week-old golden retriever joined us. Little Lucca Bean rapidly evolved through Lanky Lucca Bean into String Bean and now into an adult with an attribute Macy never did have, a sense of humour. On her first trip to France my newest dog will be renamed French Bean. Now that her adult personality is apparent it's safe to say that Bean will be a much safer dog to go travelling with. While Macy indoors had a bit of a personality bypass, outdoors she was the most excitingly fearless and confident dog I've ever lived with. Bean joyously charges off into the distance but soon after always returns. She values close companionship. If I can assure myself that I can safely protect her from all those unpleasant Mediterranean parasites, I'm thinking of taking her on a casual journey around Old Europe.

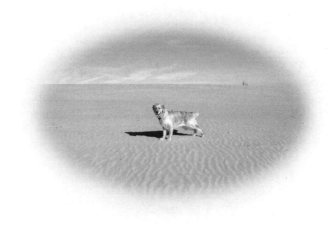

BIBLIOGRAPHY

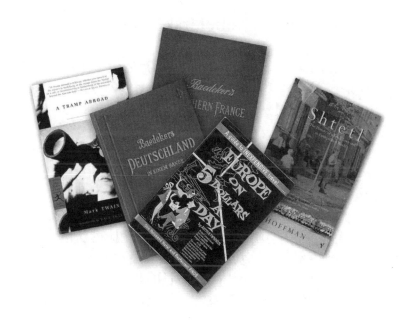

Animals My Adventure. Lutz Heck, Methuen & Co Ltd, London, 1954

Aurochs: Le retour . . . d'une supercherie nazie. Piotr Daszkiewicz & Jean Aikhenbaum, *H.S.T.E.S.* Paris, 1999

Baedeker's Austria-Hungary. Leipzig, 1911

Baedeker's Autoguide Benelux. Stuttgart, 1958

Baedeker's Belgium and Holland. Leipzig, 1888

Baedeker's Belgium and Holland. Leipzig, 1910

Baedeker's Northern France. Leipzig, 1899

Baedeker's Northern Germany. Leipzig, 1925

Baedeker's Northern Italy. Leipzig, 1913

Baedeker's Rhine. Leipzig, 1900

Baedeker's Touring Guide Italy. Freiburg, 1962

The Baltic Revolution. Anatol Lieven, Yale University Press, New Haven, 1993

Birds of Europe. Lars Jonsson, A & C Black Ltd., London, 1992

The Book of Åland. Ålands Landskapsstyrelse, Mariehamn, 2000

The Carniolan Bee. Cebelarski Musej, Radovljica, 2003

Dragonflies and Damselflies of Britain and Northern Europe. Bob Gibbons, Country Life Books, Twickenham, 1986

The Encyclopedia of Wild Flowers. John Akeroyd, Parragon, Bath, 1999

Europe: A History. Norman Davies, Oxford University Press, London, 1996

L'Europe en Automobile, Guide Officiel De L'A.I.A.C.R., Edition 1938. Zurich, 1938

Europe on $5 a Day. Arthur Frommer, Arthur Frommer Inc., New York, 1964

European Phrase Book. Dorling Kindersley, London, 2003

Field Guide to Outdooor Gotland. Jens-Henrik Kloth & Ulf Loven, Gotlands Fornsals Forlag, Visby, 2002

Frontiers. Adam Nicolson, Weidenfeld & Nicolson, London, 1985

National Parks Europe. Endat Group Ltd, Stirling, 2000

The Potato. Larry Zuckerman, North Point Press, New York, 1999

Shtetl. Eva Hoffman, Vintage, London, 1999

The Summer Book. Tove Jansson, Sort of Books, London, 2003

A Tramp Abroad. Mark Twain, Modern Library, Random House, London, 2003

Trees and Bushes of Europe. Oleg Polunin, Oxford University Press, London, 1976

Where to Watch Birds in Eastern Europe. Gerard Gorman, Hamlyn Ltd., London, 1994

Wild Herbs of Britain and Europe. Jacques de Sloover & Matine Goossens, David & Charles, London, 1994

The Year of the Hare. Arto Paasilinna, Peter Owen Publishers, London, 1995